Why You Should Read This Book

In the medical world, the FDA and drug companies define a side effect as *rare* if it occurs less often than in one in a hundred patients. But some side effects are so terrible that even if they occur in only one in a thousand, or ten thousand, or even as little as one in a hundred thousand people, they cannot be dismissed and ignored as "rare."

The drug companies would have you believe that side effects with the fluroquinolone antibiotics Cipro, Levaquin, Avelox, Factive, Floxin, and Norflox are rare. They are not, and sometimes they are severe and long lasting, or as the FDA finally admits, "permanent." This book contains many such cases, described by the patients themselves, that prove the FDA's point about the severity of the reactions to this group of drugs.

The FDA itself has received nearly 50,000 unique case reports in which the only likely culprit is one of these drugs. Yet 50,000 case reports received since 1998 are not many in comparison to the 30 *billion* of these antibiotics prescribed each year to patients in America. So the FDA's numbers are only the tip of a mammoth iceberg. The FDA's own studies have proven it identifies only five percent or fewer of actual reactions that occur with prescription drugs. Thus, once again the FDA has underestimated the likely actual count of perhaps as many as 500 thousand severe reactions to fluoroquinolones or perhaps far more. And because many doctors don't read the FDA's dire warnings about the risks, they have little knowledge about these fluoroquinolone toxicity syndromes and provide little support to patients who come to them desperately seeking assistance.

That is why this book has been written, and why Dr. Cohen has worked since 2001 to offer legitimate, evidence-based ideas for the prevention (highly possible) and treatment (sometimes possible) of this medical catastrophe that has persisted in the United States for twenty-eight years, and even longer in other countries.

When the FDA contacted Dr. Cohen in 2004 about their plan for the first major warnings about fluoroquinolones, they asked him if the people he had spoken to seemed credible. He said yes, they seemed very credible. Four years later, the FDA wrote its first black box warning on fluoroquinolones' labels. Unfortunately, today these warnings seem to go unnoticed. Hopefully, this book might be a wake-up call for more people—doctors and patients alike—to know what potential dangers there are in these commonly prescribed medications—and tell people that there are safer alternative options available.

WHAT YOU MUST KNOW ABOUT
THE HIDDEN DANGERS OF ANTIBIOTICS

JAY S. COHEN, MD

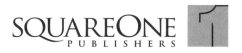

SQUAREONE
PUBLISHERS

EDITOR: Ally Cirruzzo
COVER DESIGNER: Jeannie Tudor
TYPESETTER: Gary A. Rosenberg

The information and advice contained in this book are based upon the research and experiences of the authors. They are not intended as a substitute for consulting with your physician or other healthcare provider. The publisher and authors are not responsible for any adverse effects or consequences resulting from the use of any of the information or suggestions presented in this book. All matters pertaining to your physical health should be supervised by a healthcare professional who can provide medical care that is tailored to meet individual needs.

Square One Publishers
115 Herricks Road
Garden City Park, NY 11040
(516) 535-2010 • (877) 900-BOOK
www.squareonepublishers.com

Library of Congress Cataloging-in-Publication Data

Names: Cohen, Jay S., author.
Title: What you must know about the hidden dangers of antibiotics : how the side effects of six popular antibiotics can destroy your health / Dr. Jay S. Cohen.
Description: Garden City Park, NY : Square One Publishers, [2018] | Includes bibliographical references and index.
Identifiers: LCCN 2017058348 | ISBN 9780757004698 (paperback)
Subjects: LCSH: Antibiotics—Side effects—Popular works.
Classification: LCC RM267 .C59 2018 | DDC 615.3/29—dc23

Printed in the United States of America

10   9   8   7   6   5   4   3   2

Contents

To the thousands of people seriously injured,
sometimes for years, by Cipro, Levaquin, or
one of the four other fluoroquinolone antibiotics.

Open Letter to
the Senate Committee
on Health, Education & Labor

Dear Senators:

Serious adverse reactions to fluoroquinolone antibiotics (FQs) have been reported in medical journals and to the FDA since the 1980s. Although the FDA has increased the warnings on these drugs, my analysis of the data shows that reports continue to climb in number. As of February 2014, approximately 45,000 individual cases of fluoroquinolone toxicity have been reported. And, as studies have proven, the FDA receives reports of only one to 5 percent of the actual numbers of adverse reactions that occur.

I have been following these medications for sixteen years and have evaluated in person or by telephone consultation more than 500 people injured by FQs. In 2001, I published an article, "Peripheral Neuropathy with Fluoroquinolone Antibiotics" in the peer-reviewed journal, *Annals of Pharmacotherapy*. This article described forty-five cases of neurological symptoms such as tingling, numbness, burning pain, twitching, and/or weakness. Moreover, 93 percent of agitation, impaired cognitive function, intractable insomnia, hallucinations, psychosis, acute manic episodes, joint or muscle pain, or tendon rupture. In many cases, toxicities also involved the cardiovascular and gastrointestinal systems, skin, and sight or hearing. Overall, 90 percent of my subjects experienced toxicity to multiple body systems, hence I have coined the term: *fluoroquinolone toxicity syndrome* (FTS).

Of greatest concern, the majority of my cases had lasted more than one to two years and were ongoing. These severe, long-term reactions occurred in a generally young and healthy population. The average patient was forty-two, many of them athletes. In fact, top athletic organizations now warn athletes to avoid treatment in FQs. Because of the impaired healing seen in severe FTS patients, we have long suspected genetic injury from FQs. These drugs were designed to injure the genetic structure of bacteria and thereby kill them, and they are very efficient in doing so. However, testing was never performed to ensure that FQs do indeed injure human DNA. Further study on this must now be undertaken.

There is no doubt that fluoroquinolones are important medications that help many thousands of people each year, but the indiscriminate prescribing of these highly potent "big gun" antibiotics for everyday minor infections such as sinusitis, sore throats, or bladder infections is unnecessary and medically unsafe. Medical authorities have repeatedly denounced the overuse of FQs. In my forty-plus years in pharmaco-vigilance, FQs surpass Vioxx and thalidomide in the degree of permanent harm done.

FDA warnings currently describe many of the adverse effects of FQs. Recently the FDA has finally acknowledged that FQs can cause perma-nent injury. However, FDA warnings do not adequately describe FTS syndrome, so doctors do not consider FTS a possible culprit for patients' symptoms. Instead, they waste valuable time and order expensive test-ing for rare neurologic or rheumatologic disorders while discontinuing or dismissing patients who are suffering severely from FTS. The warnings must be improved and the word about FTS must be spread nationally and worldwide. It can start with you.

Sincerely,
Jay S. Cohen, M.D.

Introduction

Suppose you develop a bladder or sinus infection and go to your doctor. Let's say your doctor does the right thing by informing you fully, saying, "Cipro is the best drug for this problem. However, drugs like Cipro are believed to cause more than 55,000 serious, sometimes disabling, sometimes permanent reactions each year. Do you still want to take it?" Would you say, "Yes, please?" Not likely. Yet, Cipro and other antibiotics just like it are prescribed to patients every day, often for minor afflictions that do not warrant the use of such a powerful drug.

Introduced in 1987 as the first oral medication of its kind, Cipro, or by its generic name, ciprofloxacin, belongs to a class of drugs known as *fluoroquinolone antibiotics.* Fluoroquinolones (FQs) are particularly potent drugs that are used to treat many different types of infections. However, they are also known for causing debilitating, long-lasting side effects. Despite this alarming fact, fluoroquinolones are one of the most commonly prescribed drugs in America.

A NATION IN PANIC

On September 18th, 2001, just a week after the terrorist attacks on the World Trade Center, five envelopes containing a strange granular substance were mailed to each major news source in America. One month later, an employee at American Media, Inc. died of inhalation anthrax, a rare but serious bacterial infection in the lungs. His death was closely followed by the discovery of more letters contaminated with what was determined to be a potent strain of anthrax spores. The nation, still reeling from 9/11, went into hysteria. Over the course of the months that followed, a total of five people died and many more were afflicted with anthrax in a mysterious case of bioterrorism committed against American civilians.

When the United States Centers for Disease Control (CDC) recommended Cipro as a preventative measure for anthrax exposure, I was concerned. I had spent two years collecting data, writing and rewriting, and then shepherding my article, "Peripheral Neuropathy Associated with Fluoroquinolone Antibiotics," toward publication. It wasn't easy. Several of the peer reviewers didn't like what I was saying in the article and tried to block its approval.

Fortunately, the publisher stood firm and set the date for publication to December 2001. After the anthrax scare in October, the publisher and I felt the information was urgently needed when Cipro became a household name and people began taking or hoarding it without medical basis. Cipro's downsides weren't widely known then, even among doctors. Yet, many of the forty-five subjects of my study were injured or disabled years after taking Cipro, suffering from neurological, musculoskeletal, psychiatric, and cardiac reactions to the drug.

THE PRESS RELEASE

The press release accompanying my article, "Peripheral Neuropathy Associated with Fluoroquinolone Antibiotics," appeared on October 22, 2001:

> Adverse effects associated with the use of ciprofloxacin (Cipro) and other fluoroquinolone antibiotics are not always benign. Not infrequently, they can be severe and permanently disabling, and they may occur following just one or a few doses, according to a study posted on The Annals of Pharmacotherapy Web site today.

The article described forty-five cases of FQ toxicity involving the peripheral nervous system, such as tingling, numbness, weakness, burning pain, twitching, or spasms. In addition, 93 percent of the subjects sustained adverse side effects involving other systems: 78 percent experienced central nervous system (CNS) symptoms such as dizziness, agitation, impaired cognitive function, intractable insomnia, or hallucinations; and 73 percent reported musculoskeletal symptoms such as joint or muscle pain or tendon rupture. In many cases, toxicities also involved the cardiovascular and gastrointestinal systems, skin, and sight or hearing.

The age of subjects in my survey ranged between eleven to sixty-eight years old, with an average age of forty-two. The great majority of the cases of FQ toxicity were severe, lasting three months in 71 percent and exceeding one year in 58 percent of cases. In 62 percent of these cases, subjects had no other medical disorder except an infection (sinusitis, prostatitis, or urinary infection) that led to FQ treatment. In other words, these people were mostly young, healthy individuals— until FQ therapy.

The media jumped on my article and wrote about it in newspapers and magazines. My telephone rang a lot. I spent a few minutes on NPR's Morning Edition with Bob Edwards. Within days, the CDC announced it was dropping Cipro as the favored antibiotic for anthrax exposure and now recommended much safer antibiotics, such as doxycycline.

ANTHRAX OR CIPRO?

I wish I could say that was the end of it, but it was just the beginning. Six months later the *Washington Post* carried a story, "Anthrax Patients' Ailments Linger." The story described symptoms such as fatigue, exhaustion, joint pain, and memory problems lingering in some postal workers. The article pointed its finger at anthrax exposure, but I suspected many of the cases were from Cipro toxicity.

Five days later, the United Press International posted "Anthrax Ills Mirror Cipro Side Effects" on its website:

Doctors treating several survivors of last year's anthrax attacks describe a continuing set of symptoms that are similar to reported side effects of the main drug used to treat them. Side effects include joint pain, fatigue, confusion, difficulty concentrating, and memory loss.

"They all fit, right down the line," said Dr. Jay S. Cohen. He said Cipro and other fluoroquinolone antibiotics are well-documented as sometimes causing psychiatric and neurological side effects, as well as musculoskeletal problems. Doctors following these cases do not know whether the problems suffered by the handful of anthrax survivors are related to Cipro or from anthrax.

"It is an interesting possibility," said Dr. Mark Galbraith, an infectious disease specialist in Virginia who is treating one survivor. He discontinued Cipro for his fifty-nine year old patient after two weeks because of a rash and painful joints. Months later, joint pain and difficulty persist. The CDC acknowledged that a percentage of patients did not continue their Cipro because of side effects including joint pain, dizziness, nausea, fatigue, or diarrhea.

"A lot of people did stop taking it," said American Postal Workers Union spokeswoman Sally Daridow. The organization has asked

Congress to investigate how Cipro and other antibiotics might affect workers long-term.

Congress never did, so in 2004 I sent a letter to Congressman Rush Holt of New Jersey, asking for an investigation. Nothing materialized.

In December 2001, the *American Spectator* published the following in *Ben Stein's Diary*:

> We [Stein and another person] talked for a long time about the anthrax threat in D.C. and then about the medicine of choice, Cipro, that's being prescribed for it. Just by fate, I had been given Cipro a few weeks before and had suffered simply horrible, dreadful, unbelievably bad psychological side effects: dread, suicidal thinking, panic. In fact, I had the first real panic attacks I had endured since I stopped taking benzo-diazepines about twelve years before. I had been mystified about what was causing them until I looked up Cipro in the paperback edition of the *Physicians' Desk Reference*, only to find that high among the list of side effects are "abnormal fear" and "dread." My doctor pooh-poohed these effects, but when I stopped taking the Cipro, the effects disappeared pronto.

The suddenness of Stein's reaction and its severity are typical of many accounts of FQ toxicity. In my study, 58 percent of patients developed reactions within three days of starting a FQ. Also, 70 percent had symptoms like Stein's involving the central nervous system, such as severe agitation, panic, impaired thinking, hallucinations, suicidal ideation, insomnia, and "brain fog." Typically, Stein's doctor dismissed the reaction, although there were no other credible explanations for his symptoms. His doctor's ignorance wasn't anything unusual, either. At the same time, the health editor of a national magazine wrote that a thirty-day course of ciprofloxacin "wouldn't cause a healthy adult much harm."

Fortunately, Stein's toxic reaction cleared quickly. He was one of the lucky ones.

THOUSANDS SEEKING HELP

After publishing "Peripheral Neuropathy Associated with Fluoroquinolone Antibiotics," I began to receive letters and emails. This one arrived a few months later, in early 2002, from a bioengineer at a local biotech company:

I am a thirty year old female with no medical problems before I was given Cipro for a suspected urinary tract infection in March 2002, though my culture came back clean later. I took Cipro for only three days and have been having muscle, tendon, and joint pain since. I was so devastated last week while reading emails from an adverse drug reactions forum, since most of them are saying that the symptoms would go on for years and years. I almost cried on the way home from work as I was driving by the beach and worrying I might never be able to run along the shore again. What's troublesome about this whole situation is the lack of awareness of the doctor about this problem. Like many cases in your paper, my doctor too dismissed the idea that my symptoms have anything to do with Cipro and no one warned me of anything before I took it. I do wish that, one day down the road, people could at least get a warning from their doctors before they took the medicine.

I felt badly because I had little help to offer her. Today I could offer many suggestions, although still there is no well-proven remedy.

"At least you listen to me," she said to me, "At least you believe me. You understand the harm these drugs can do."

THE PROBLEM WITH FLUOROQUINOLONES

Since 2001, I have consulted with people from the United States and Canada who've been "floxed," the term used by people badly injured by FQs, although we rightly could use the word "poisoned." Over the last fifteen years, I have spoken with approximately 500 such people who've become seriously injured—often times to the point of disability—after using FQs.

"Only 500 cases—what's the big fuss, Cohen?" you might ask. The number today is about 50,000 cases reported to the FDA, and according to RxISK.org, 79,000 reports and 1,700 deaths with Cipro alone, and the FDA's number may likely be ten or twenty times higher. This is the definition of an epidemic, and it is wholly man-made.

The problem is, it is unlikely you'd ever get an accurate description of FQ's toxicities from most doctors. Studies show that only 10 to 25 percent of patients receive adequate warnings from their doctors about the drugs they are prescribed. This means that 75 to 90 percent do not. And if many doctors are unaware of the extent and severity of FQ reactions, how could they provide you with an adequate warning in the first place?

It is not an exaggeration for me to say that the development of penicillin and subsequent antibiotics are among the top achievements in the history of medicine. Because of these wonder drugs, the top causes of death in the early twentieth century, pneumonia and tuberculosis, are no longer feared. Drugs can perform miracles, and I prescribe them every day in my practice. Yet with all due respect to the good things FQs accomplish—they can indeed be life-saving—the number and severity of FQ toxicities are unacceptable.

WHAT'S IN THIS BOOK

Part 1 of this book, "The Problem," will introduce you to fluoroquinolones and their potential for destruction. Chapter 1 addresses the issue at hand: fluoroquinolone antibiotics are commonly prescribed but hazardous drugs. You will learn how and why doctors seem to have overlooked the dangers of these popular drugs for almost thirty years. Chapters 2 through 4 discuss how fluoroquinolone toxicity syndrome affects the tendons, joints, and bones; the central and peripheral nervous systems; and other parts of the body, including the heart, gut, and brain. Finally, Chapter 5 will explain how quinolones are damaging to DNA.

The second part of this book, "What We Must Do Now," starts by explaining the various kinds of medications, supplements, and other treatments that can be used to fight fluoroquinolone toxicity syndrome. Chapter 8 discusses at length how the mineral magnesium does wonders for treating FTS and includes a guide to using magnesium to treat toxicity symptoms. Chapter 9 focuses on three other types of medications—N-acetylcysteine, zinc, and vitamin E—which have been scientifically proven to combat FTS. Chapter 10 lists a number of treatments that many sufferers of FTS have used to treat their symptoms. The final chapter in the book outlines the action steps I have devised in order to stop fluoroquinolone toxicity and gives pointers on what we can do going forward.

This book is not about bad drugs that must be banned. It is about good drugs that have saved hundreds of thousands of people, but have also severely injured tens of thousands of others, sometimes permanently. Doctors remain poorly informed, dismissing people who have become seriously injured after taking fluoroquinolones. Currently there are no scientifically proven treatments for what I call *fluoroquinolone toxicity syndrome*, or FTS. My goal in writing this book is to shed much-needed light on a terrible medical problem that persists today, and to also encourage efforts toward finding more effective solutions.

The FQ tragedy ranks among the worst in history of modern medicine in terms of numbers, pain, and disability. Unfortunately, the tragedy will continue until appropriate FQ use is clearly defined and limited to serious or life-threatening medical disorders by the drug companies and FDA; patients are fully informed about the possible toxicities of FQs before they are prescribed them by their doctors; doctors prescribe FQs only when there is a legitimate, proven reason for their use; and doctors correctly identify FTS reactions and report them to the FDA. The poisoning of healthy people by FQs has to stop. And we can start accomplishing this now.

PART ONE

The Problem

1

The Most Popular Antibiotic in America

Antibiotics are one of the most frequently prescribed medications today. They fight a wide array of minor and serious infections alike by killing or injuring bacteria in the body. Most people are prescribed an antibiotic at some point in their lives. They are an incredibly useful advancement of modern medicine and help many people—when they are prescribed judiciously.

Quinolones are a particularly powerful class of *broad spectrum* antibiotics, meaning they are effective against a wide range of bacteria. The majority of quinolones in use today are *fluoroquinolones*, or FQs, named for the fluorine atom in their chemical structure. Antibiotics such as penicillin, erythromycin, and tetracycline are called *bacteriostatic* because they prevent bacteria from multiplying until they die. In contrast, FQs are *bactericidal*, meaning that they kill bacteria outright. They accomplish this by attaching to bacterial DNA and preventing its duplication, killing bacteria more quickly than the bacteriostatic antibiotics.

Fluoroquinolones are used to fight many types of infections involving the lungs, brain, bones, joints, gastrointestinal tract, or prostate. Because they are so powerful, FQs are considered "big guns" among antibiotics available today. They became very popular very quickly, tripling in prescriptions filled between 1995 and 2002, and have been further increasing in popularity ever since. In recent years, FQs have become the most prescribed group of antibiotics in America.

FLUOROQUINOLONE TOXICITY SYNDROME

Fluoroquinolones are associated with a number of serious, often debilitating side effects. The most common are damage to the central and peripheral nervous systems and tendon ruptures and other injuries to

Currently Available Fluoroquinolone Antibiotics

- Avelox (moxifloxacin), approved 1999
- Cipro (ciprofloxacin), approved 1987
- Factive (gemifloxacin), approved 2003
- Floxin (ofloxacin), approved 1990
- Levaquin (levofloxacin), approved 1996
- Norflox (norfloxacin), approved 1986

According to the FDA, approximately 23 million office patients received prescriptions for FQs in 2011. Additional millions received FQs in hospitals. Nearly 70 percent of FQ prescriptions are for ciprofloxacin, the generic form of Cipro. Levaquin and its generic, levofloxacin, accounted for about 22 percent, and Avelox (moxifloxacin) for 7 percent of FQ sales. Norfloxacin, ofloxacin, and gemifloxacin account for less than one percent of FQ prescriptions.

connective tissue. The adverse effects from FQs are often the result of a serious condition myself and the many affected refer to as *fluoroquinolone toxicity syndrome,* or FTS. Despite FDA-issued warnings of the dangers of FQs, thousands of people continue to suffer from FTS.

Injury from a fluoroquinolone antibiotic was first reported in 1972. It involved the original, first-generation FQ, nalidixic acid. The report by Bailey, Natale, and Linton read:

A twenty-two year old woman with a series of multiple bladder infections and a kidney infection experienced visual distortions, intense brightness from lights, visual hallucinations and became delirious soon after being placed on nalidixic acid. The symptoms disappeared quickly after the medication was stopped. Later that year, the kidney infection returned and one day after again receiving nalidixic acid, the woman developed severe joint pain, swelling, redness and other pain. These symptoms began in the feet and ankles, then spread to her knees, hands, wrists, elbows and right shoulder. Soon after, her prior visual disturbances returned. Other symptoms included nightmares, weakness, sudden crying and loss of appetite. Pain limited her ability to move, and many joints were swollen and hot. Finally, the nalidixic acid was discontinued, and over the next seventeen days she recovered.

Note that this person's adverse reaction was not limited to one area or system of her body. It wasn't a typical adverse reaction like nausea, dizziness, headache, or constipation. This reaction exhibited neurological, musculoskeletal, psychiatric, and visual aspects. It was severe, painful, long-lasting, and temporarily disabling.

At the time his letter was published, Dr. Bailey contacted the manufacturer and learned it had received "about a dozen reports of side effects relevant to the joints." Thus, as far back as 1972, serious adverse side effects of fluoroquinolones were seen and reported. Eleven years later, in 1983, Dr. Bailey published another incident of joint pain from a FQ. Then, in 1988, McEwan and Davey published a case report of bilateral Achilles tendinitis induced by fluoroquinolones and also noted that by late 1987, fourteen other cases of FQ-related musculoskeletal adverse events, including one tendon rupture, had been reported to United Kingdom officials. They also noted that in France, sixty-three incidents of joint, muscle, and/or tendon pain had been reported.

Also in 1987, Cipro, the first modern FQ, was approved in the United States with no major warnings of its potential dangers.

NEEDLESS PRESCRIPTIONS

As the most prescribed antibiotics in America, FQs get prescribed inappropriately a lot. Many people with whom I've consulted were prescribed FQs needlessly. Minor infections like bladder or sinus infections are rarely life-threatening and should be treated initially not with big guns or big risks, but with safer antibiotics, which are usually sufficient. Some FQs are prescribed without any evidence that an infection exists in the first place. Remember, antibiotics are only useful for killing bacteria. They are useless against viruses, allergies, inflammation, or other causes of discomfort or pain.

Sore throats are usually benign and transitory. They are typically caused by viruses, which antibiotics are useless against. Doctors have known this for decades, and yet one of the most common uses of antibiotics—and FQs in particular—is for treating sore throats. In 2001, the *Journal of the American Medical Association* (JAMA) published a study that measured the overuse of antibiotics by doctors treating sore throats. The researchers swabbed the throats of people complaining of soreness and cultured the bacteria for streptococcal bacterial infection, or strep throat. They found only 5 to 17 percent had strep and actually required antibiotic therapy. Nevertheless, doctors had prescribed antibiotics to 73 percent of patients. And although several safer antibiotics can be used for strep throat, FQs were often prescribed by the doctors. Imagine, getting FTS because of a simple virus that didn't warrant antibiotic treatment in the first place, and certainly not a big gun FQ.

The first sentence of a 2005 article in the journal *Expert Opinion on Drug Safety* states, "Fluoroquinolones are the most potent antibiotics in clinical use today. Increasingly, these drugs are being prescribed for relatively benign infections and for new categories of patients, including pediatric patients. As their use becomes more frequent, so will the adverse effects." How true. Here's an example from H.K., age thirty-six, who was previously healthy:

> I was prescribed Levaquin for a sore throat. I took 500 mg on April 15, 2014, in both the morning and evening. That night, I had insomnia, hallucinations, nightmares, and a rapid heartbeat. I then took one more 500 mg dose the next morning. An hour later I had dizziness, vertigo, panic attack, very rapid heartbeat, and strange, disquieting thoughts. I went to my primary care physician. She prescribed Xanax. She figured the Levaquin would be out of my system in forty-eight hours, but I didn't see any improvement. A week later, she prescribed Lexapro for anxiety and depression. I took that for six days but continued to worsen: depression, loss of appetite, nervousness, anxiety attacks. We agreed to discontinue the Lexapro. I have only seen limited improvement overall since April 29th, three days after I stopped Lexapro. For fifteen days I had to take Xanax to fall asleep. I would wake up with palpitations, anxiety, disruptive thoughts, and tingling and burning in my arms. My symptoms would come in waves. Bad in the morning, improvement during the day, then worst at night. I also noticed after I ate I would start feeling the anxiety. Most doctors I have talked to say they haven't heard of Levaquin having such a reaction.

It is widely known among experts that fluoroquinolone antibiotics are "big guns," that is, they are among our most powerful antibiotics. The authors of a 2002 article in *American Family Physician* state, "The new fluoroquinolones are rarely first line agents and should be employed judiciously." Too often, they aren't.

WHO IS AT RISK?

The FDA defines the "at-risk groups" for FTS as those sixty or older, those with organ transplants or undergoing renal dialysis, and those given FQs while receiving steroids or NSAIDs. This warning has been issued by the FDA, sent to all doctors, and included in all black-box warnings for FQs on package inserts and other written materials from the drug manufacturers. Despite the FDA's intentions to inform, these black-box warnings present a problem in reverse. Many doctors read the warning and interpret it as meaning that people without these risk factors have little possibility of developing FTS. I've heard doctors say that FQs have few side effects except in the groups the FDA has named.

This interpretation is incorrect and misleading. Quite the opposite, our data show that many more people below the age of sixty have experienced FTS than people above this age. I have had doctors, after prescribing FQs thoughtlessly and incorrectly, state in court that people below sixty are not susceptible to FTS. In other words, doctors turn the warning around to their own advantage. They reason that, if the FDA says people older than sixty are most at risk, then people below sixty must have little risk. This is inaccurate. The warnings don't say that at all. Yet, that's how doctors interpret it, especially when they are being sued—and when they are being defended by a shrewd attorney.

This warning needs to be rewritten in order to not mislead doctors and other healthcare providers and their patients. The average age of reports to the FDA is fifty-five. In my experience, there are many more young people afflicted with FTS than elderly. Perhaps this vulnerability of young people reflects the increased risk in athletes and other physically active populations. Another at-risk group may be younger, sexually active women who are prone to frequent urinary tract infections. FQs should also be used with utmost caution in women of childbearing age, especially those who are attempting to become pregnant. FDA warnings advise pregnant women or those attempting to become pregnant to avoid FQs. So should women who are breastfeeding, because FQs can pass in breast milk.

The Mayo Clinic doctors add, "Until more is known, caution should be exercised in the prescription of fluoroquinolone antibiotics when other classes of antibiotics are available." In most cases of urinary or sinus infections, other classes of effective antibiotics are often an alternative choice. FQs may be the best choice for very serious infections involving lungs, kidneys, or prostates, but always be sure to ask the doctor why he or she is prescribing a FQ and if there are other, safer alternatives.

I have listed some of the Mayo Clinic's recommendations verbatim because their descriptions of the origin of FTS injuries and the guidelines for the safe use of FQs are accurate. Since so many doctors are unaware of the dire risks of these drugs, you may find the Mayo Clinic's guidelines helpful in discussing your concerns about FTS with your doctors. Because so few FTS victims have received proper warnings when prescribed FQs, the Mayo Clinic article appropriately ends with this: "Patients should always be counseled regarding the risk associated with fluoroquinolones, even when they are prescribed according to standard recommendations."

FQ Use in Children

FQs should not be prescribed for children and adolescents unless absolutely necessary. Studies of FQs used in young rats and beagles indicated that the drugs caused extensive damage to their developing cartilage. In 2006, the Committee of Infectious Diseases of the American Academy of Pediatrics recommended that FQs be restricted to "situations in which there is no safe and effective alternative to treat an infection cause by multi-drug resistant bacteria, or to provide oral therapy when parenteral [intravenous] therapy is not feasible and no other effective oral agent is available." The FDA makes exceptions only for serious infections that are not sensitive to or have not responded to other antibiotics. Despite these restrictions on FQ use in children, in 2002 there were 520,000 prescriptions filled in the United States for patients younger than eighteen years old.

Nevertheless, there has been some debate in the medical literature about whether the evidence supports restricting FQ use in youngsters. Two studies have found no evidence that FQs cause a greater frequency of musculoskeletal disorders than other antibiotics. Yet in a study that compared adverse effects in several thousand children given Levaquin in comparison to adverse events with non-FQ antibiotics, there was a greater incidence of musculoskeletal problems with Levaquin. These adverse effects included joint pain, arthritis, tendon pain, or impaired walking. Other studies have also shown that FQs produce a higher frequency of musculoskeletal problems in children than other antibiotics. My view is that the restrictions on FQs in children are correct and should be extended to everyone. FQs should not be used as first choice drugs for any condition unless other antibiotics are ineffective or laboratory testing shows that the bacteria are sensitive only to FQs. In other words, *use only when necessary!*

EXCESSIVE DOSING

Drug companies are required to provide information on dosage. This includes antibiotics, for which manufacturers often recommend dosages that vary on the severity or location of the infections. Some doctors, however, learn a specific dosage and provide this to all patients no matter the type of the infection. This leads to overmedication and unnecessary risks. Prescribing the proper dosage of a medication to a patient is one of the most basic tenets of competent medical care.

For example, I have received many cases in which doctors prescribed 500 mg of Cipro twice daily for five days to treat a patient with a mild urinary tract infection. The proper dosage of Cipro for a mild UTI is 250 mg twice daily for three days. These people received double the recommended dosage, as well as receiving it for five days instead of only three. The result was that rather than receiving a total of 1,500 mg of Cipro, they received 5,000—more than triple the needed amount. Side effects are a function of dosage. The higher the dosage, the higher the risk. It's no different than with alcohol or coffee: excessive amounts cause greater problems.

Some people I've spoken with had none of the hallmarks of a urinary infection, but the doctors prescribed a FQ anyway. Doctors are given the right to prescribe drugs when they have a suspicion of a problem even if the evidence is lacking. But why prescribe a big gun FQ with serious risks instead of other effective and safe antibiotics for a mild UTI? It doesn't make sense logically, medically, or ethically.

PDR-Recommended Doses of Cipro for Urinary Tract Infections

Acute or Uncomplicated: 250 mg twice daily for three days.

Mild to Moderate: 250 mg twice daily for fourteen days.

Severe or Complicated: 500 mg twice daily for fourteen days.

For more than fifty years, medical school textbooks and medical journal articles have made the point that proper dosing of medications is a fundamental tenet of quality and ethical medical practices. *Goodman and Gilman's The Pharmacological Basis of Therapeutics* states, "The right dose differentiates a poison and a remedy." Medications do wonders for sick patients, but can cause more harm than good when prescribed irresponsibly. Pharmacists have a saying: "Right patient, right drug, right dosage." They have it for a reason. It is the responsibility of every pharmacist and doctor to avoid overmedicating patients. Higher doses always bring greater risks. Sometimes no harm occurs, but sometimes it does, and with FQs it can destroy a person's life.

LACK OF TRAINING OR LACK OF INTEREST?

Why do doctors prescribe FQs so needlessly and, at times, irresponsibly? And why do they do so against the advice of FQ manufacturers, the FDA, and experts on antibiotic use? Don't doctors read the letters sent to them by the manufacturers, as ordered by the FDA, warning of the severe adverse effects of these drugs? Don't doctors see the black-box warnings posted on materials such as package inserts and PDR descriptions? Black-box warnings are the strongest warnings the FDA issues about the most severe medication side effects. Aren't doctors paying attention?

In March 2014, I was told the following by Bill H.:

> My son Richard was a healthy and athletic twenty-year-old junior at college when he developed signs of a sinus infection. The doctor prescribed Zithromax (azithromycin), but Richard was allergic to it. The doctor then prescribed Levaquin. After two doses, Richard developed severe muscle and joint pains, stomach pain, and extreme exhaustion. Other side effects soon emerged, including anxiety, insomnia, nerve pains, and many others. I estimate he developed about 70 percent of the many side effects listed in Levaquin. The doctor said the drug would have already been out of Richard's system, so it couldn't possibly be causing these problems. Another doctor said he had never heard of such a reaction to Levaquin. Finally, I began searching on the internet and found extensive information and many horror stories about Levaquin's side effects. By the way, we took a Levaquin package insert to the doctor, and he refused to look at the warnings.

I know there are many doctors who try hard to treat patients safely and effectively. However, it is disappointing and discouraging when I hear stories of people with obvious FQ reactions going to doctor after doctor and being told the symptoms cannot possibly be related to the antibiotics. To say that a side effect cannot persist after the drug has exited the human system is total ignorance of basic pharmacology. The entire field of toxicology is predicated on the fact that many drugs have toxic effects that last long after the drugs have exited the human system. For example, overuse of the drugs Tylenol and Lipitor can lead to liver failure—the drugs may be gone, but the liver damage can still kill you. What is so hard to understand about that?

Deep Problems in Medical Training

The future of my profession worries me when I hear about doctors refusing to look at anything from the internet that people with fluoroquinolone toxicity syndrome bring to them, even from reliable sources like the FDA or websites like the Mayo Clinic, Johns Hopkins, or other top-flight universities. How have we gotten to a point where bringing information to the doctor is a bad thing? Doctors are supposed to work cooperatively with their patients, not defensively or antagonistically.

"I have worked for the drug industry for twenty-five years, and I am now shocked that none of my doctors bothered to simply research the possible origin of my problems," R.W., a fifty-two-year-old woman with FTS from Avelox told me in February 2014. "You'd think they would at least want to check it out. The information is right there in the package insert, PDR, or whatever source of prescription information they use!"

In my day, medical education was mainly a rote process: this disease, that treatment, with hardly any training in researching the conditions we would see or treatments we would recommend. I hope medical education has improved since then, but so far I've seen few signs of it. Patients of all ages tell me they often run into brick walls with their doctors regarding FQs, no matter the doctor's age or gender.

At the same time, I realize that the people who contact me are the ones injured by FQs and doing poorly, and therefore are dissatisfied with their doctors. I hope that the majority of people injured by FQs are receiving good, compassionate care. But I must add that for all the books and medical journals I've written on improving medication safety, I had heard hundreds of similar complaints from people injured by all kinds of drugs about their doctors' incompetence or defensiveness in dealing with people's side effects.

One thing is very clear to me: doctors are subtly yet systematically trained to discount or dismiss people's views. We used to talk about the natural alliance between doctors and patients. Today, doctors are taught to disdain the anecdotal information of patients, as if "anecdotal" reports are a bad thing. In fact, the FDA strongly relies on anecdotal reports about side effects to decide whether to ban a dangerous drug. And at least half of the advances of modern medication therapy have emerged from patients' personal reports of experiences, good and bad, with drugs.

One woman captured the feelings of many patients after her doctor ignored a serious reaction to FQ: "Doctors don't ask about side effects and don't want to hear about them. They would rather assume the problem is from some other cause, not the drug."

Yet most doctors are caring by nature. The problem is the lack of training in how to work with patients who are reporting serious side effects. Many doctors have never had a single course or lecture on how to effectively handle the situation. Medical students are not taught how to critically evaluate drug studies, or to examine the adequacy of a drug company's research on key issues of toxicology or proper dosing. They are not encouraged to develop enquiring minds about what their credible patients tell them and to simply develop the ability to think independently and analytically.

Patients Taking Agency

The ego-attachment of some doctors to their medications can become pathological and pernicious when patients express concern over side effects. Doctors may uncritically accept biased information from the drug companies or from their ever-present sales representatives, yet stonewall legitimate complaints from their own patients. Patients today are more knowledgeable and active than ever. They do their own research, read books and articles, and ask intelligent questions. Most of my patients are pretty smart and expect me to consider their ideas. I like patients who bother to inform themselves, and I enjoy discussing issues with them. In turn, patients appreciate doctors who listen to them, treat them as intelligent human beings, and don't dismiss them out of hand.

A fifty-one-year-old woman wrote to me, "One of the hardest things to comprehend through all of this is the ignorance of most doctors concerning these side effects." Previously healthy and athletic, she developed an infection after abdominal surgery. Her doctor prescribed her Levaquin. Within two days she began experiencing electrical sensations and numbness in her legs. Her doctors did not recognize these as Levaquin side effects, so they told her to finish the twenty-one-day prescription. By that time, she had tendinitis in her shoulder and knee, a partially torn Achilles tendon, and impaired concentration and memory. She needed crutches for three months, and after a year the tendon and memory problems persisted. Although the adverse reactions involving nerves, joints, and tendons were already well-known side effects of Levaquin, her physicians still dismissed the possibility of a drug reaction.

Dr. Raymond Woosley, vice president for the health sciences at the University of Arizona and a former chairman of pharmacology at Georgetown University, has summed it up well: "The United States society has invested in developing wondrous new pharmacologic therapies but has failed to invest adequately in their safe use." Dr. Woosley told me that he continually sought additional time to offer a more in-depth class on pharmacology for his students. The universities repeatedly turned him down.

My strong view is that doctors' dismissive attitude about side effects is a result of the dominance of the drug industry on medical education. According to the drug industry, only large, intensive studies provide knowledge, and everything else should be ignored. Doctors are taught that *evidence-based medicine,* the new standard for quality care, requires large studies. This is completely wrong. It is simply the influence of the drug industry on medical education. Objective definitions of evidence-based medicine emphasize that smaller studies, doctors' experiences, and patients' personal experiences also count as legitimate evidence. Large drug companies' studies can of course be very useful, but they are not always the end all, be all. They are often way off about medication doses, and they often miss major adverse effects. And as medical textbooks emphasize, the ultimate test is how a drug affects an individual patient.

Most of the hundreds of people I've spoken to about FQ reactions were previously healthy, active, educated, gainfully employed, and credible. To be dismissed out of hand by doctors saying, "I've never heard of such a reaction, so it cannot have been the Levaquin," (or the Cipro, Avelox, etc.) is both frustrating and alarming. I implore doctors to listen to their patients when they come in with complaints of unusual or severe reactions, just as I advise patients to advocate for themselves when they feel that something isn't right.

THE ROLE OF THE FDA

To be fair to doctors, the FDA hasn't helped them understand the extent of FQ reactions. I am a supporter of the FDA. These people tackle very difficult problems and have to make hard decisions about drugs that help some and harm others. I am glad I don't have their jobs.

But with FQs, the FDA has been playing catch-up from the start. The FDA should have recognized the potential dangers of FQs before approving them. They should have been better prepared because of the many severe problems with these drugs reported in other countries before FQs were approved here, and also seen vividly in early studies in animals. The FDA should have demanded more thorough research before approving FQs and required stronger warnings when it did. The warnings are better now, but it has taken decades to achieve. And even now the warnings are not enough to make doctors fully informed.

Even today, the warnings do not come close to conveying to doctors, pharmacists, and other healthcare professionals the full extent and depth of FTS. When doctors read or hear about tendon injuries with FQ, they assume it means a tendon or two. Doctors are completely unprepared for people with the plethora and diversity of symptoms involving so many human systems. They have no clue about the breadth and great severity of FTS. Most doctors really want to identify what is going on and help a patient with FTS. They order million-dollar workups with scores of blood tests, X-rays, MRIs, CT scans, and multiple consultations with specialists. From doctors' experiences, they assume the cause must be some unusual autoimmune or neurological or immunological disorder. Because they have never heard of FTS, they cannot conceive that a mere antibiotic reaction could possibly involve so many systems and be of such severity and tenacity.

CONCLUSION

It is the job of the FDA and drug companies to inform patients and doctors about the dangers of certain medications. Even after more than twenty-five years on the market, the warnings do not elucidate the severity of fluoroquinolone toxicity to doctors, and so doctors do not display appropriate caution or provide fair warning when prescribing FQs to their patients. Doctors can only diagnose the conditions they know. They cannot diagnose conditions they've never heard of before. And in too many cases, doctors can get frustrated and start blaming the patients by deciding it is a psychiatric problem or simply shun them. This unfortunately leaves many suffers of fluoroquinolone toxicity syndrome isolated and furthers their pain, depression, and hopelessness.

2

Toxicity in Tendons, Joints, and Bones

In the beginning of 2014, I spoke with Chris. When his sinus headache did not improve with the Z-Pack (azithromycin), the doctor prescribed him Avelox, as well as prednisone. Prednisone is a steroid commonly prescribed with an antibiotic for sinus infections because it can shrink swollen sinus membranes. However, steroids are absolutely *contraindicated* for their use with a FQ, meaning the combination of the two drugs can cause adverse effects and is therefore inadvisable. Chris did not take the prednisone because within three hours of his first Avelox pill, he experienced intense tingling in his arms and legs, pain in his back and sternum, muscle weakness, and trouble walking. He went to urgent care and was inaccurately diagnosed with an allergic reaction and given prednisone again, which he then took. His symptoms intensified: "I felt like I was going to die. I had trouble breathing. My heart was pounding. I was in severe pain. I could barely walk. Everything felt like it was going crazy in my body."

Chris's primary care doctor recognized it was a reaction to Avelox and referred him to a neurologist and rheumatologist. He had scores of blood tests, an MRI, and a CT scan. All were normal, but clearly he wasn't. None of the doctors had any suggestions for treatment.

From his reaction in September 2013 to our conversation five months later, some of Chris's symptoms had abated, but he continued to have others. Chris explained, "I still have joint pain, leg swelling, popping sensations in my joints, and tingling and electrical pain in my arms and legs. I cannot exercise and continue to have trouble sleeping." Chris's doctor probably meant well in prescribing him a combination of Avelox and prednisone, but he ended up in worse shape than he had started. Remember, he initially went to the doctor seeking treatment for a sinus headache.

Instead, he developed a whole new set of problems after becoming afflict-ed with fluoroquinolone toxicity.

INJURIES TO TENDONS

Tendons are fibrous tissues, made primarily of protein-rich collagen, that connect muscles to bones. They convey the power of muscle contractions onto bony structures, thereby moving the bones. For example, to bend your elbow, your biceps muscle contracts, the biceps tendon carries the contraction to the elbow, and your forearm bends toward your shoulder.

Healthy tendons are essential for normal voluntary movement of the body. Tendon inflammation or injury can cause pain at rest and especial-ly with use. Although Achilles rupture is the most notorious and recog-nized adverse drug event of FQs, any tendon in the body is vulnerable. Injuries to tendons of the hand, elbow, shoulder, foot, ankle, knee, thigh, and eye muscles have been reported in medical journals. I have spoken to many people whose injuries involved multiple tendons. When the inju-ry is severe and involves more than one tendon, disability often occurs. People cannot move without pain, so they restrict their motion. One man spent his first year after FQ toxicity on his couch, going into the kitchen or bathroom only when necessary.

FQ reactions impacting tendons may be brief (days or weeks), or they may last a few months, or many months or years. These injuries can affect other body systems too: central nervous system, peripheral nervous sys-tem, cardiovascular or gastrointestinal systems, skin, and so on. One man recently reported widespread tendon pain accompanied by high anxiety, insomnia, dizziness, weakness, nerve pain in his legs, and intense heart palpitations.

Risk Factors for FQ-Related Musculoskeletal Injuries

Proven Risk Factors

- Simultaneous use of corticosteroids

- Age sixty or older

- Sports activities or intense exercise

- Magnesium deficiency

- Trauma to tendons or joints

- History of organ transplantation

- End-stage kidney disease and/or dialysis

Suspected Risk Factors

- Osteoarthritis or rheumatoid arthritis
- Systemic lupus erythematosus
- Ankylosing spondylitis
- Reiter's syndrome
- Polymyalgia rheumatica

- Ulcerative colitis
- Crohn's disease
- Diabetes mellitus
- Hypothyrodism
- Hyperparathyrodism

INJURY REPORTS

Despite the many reports of tendon, joint, and muscle injuries with FQs during the 1980s, Cipro was approved in the United States with inadequate warnings of the harm the drug could do. By the early 1990s, the flow of injury reports intensified. For example, a 1992 report described a case of bilateral Achilles tendon ruptures in a person on a FQ. Achilles tendon ruptures are unusual unless from trauma (football, running, climbing, car accident). Bilateral Achilles tendon ruptures are even rarer. In this case, there was no trauma. The cause had to be something else.

Another 1992 report, "Seven Achilles Tendinitis Including Three Complicated by Rupture During Fluoroquinolone Therapy" was published in the *Journal of Rheumatology*. In 1994, a report from France described 100 cases of tendon injuries including thirty-one tendon ruptures with FQs. Also in 1994, Dr. K. Huston published a letter in the *New England Journal of Medicine* describing an eighty-five-year-old man, already on prednisone for a rheumatologic disorder, who developed a rupture of his right Achilles tendon following treatment with a FQ. Worried by what occurred, Dr. Huston added prophetically:

> Fluoroquinolone antibiotics have been associated with Achilles tendinitis and rupture in reports from Europe and New Zealand. This unusual side effect has not been widely recognized in the United States and is not mentioned in the *Physicians' Desk Reference*. Physicians should be aware of this potential complication.

We might wonder why, with so many reports, healthcare professionals in the United States were not made quickly aware of the problem. Unfortunately, in spite of its publication in top medical journals, Huston's statement made little impact. By 1997, the *Physician's Desk Reference* (PDR) did mention tendinitis in its description of Cipro, but you'd have to look hard to find it. The PDR information on Cipro occupied three entire pages of the voluminous book. Among 900 lines of information, the warning about tendon reactions comprised a barely visible five lines mentioning that inflammation, muscle pain, tendinitis, or tendon rupture could occur with Cipro. Most doctors probably never saw it.

THE REPORTS KEEP COMING

From the fourth quarter of 1997 to the fourth quarter of 2012, the FDA received 12,088 reports of individual cases of FQ-related injuries to people's musculoskeletal systems. Tendon rupture occurred in 2,141 of these 12,088 cases. Imagine, more than 2,000 people suffering tendon ruptures, muscle being ripped from bone, and often other injuries as well. Who could have imagined an antibiotic could do such damage? A tendon rupture results in extreme pain, prolonged incapacity, and in many cases, surgery and disability. As these injuries don't always heal completely, someone suffering a tendon rupture often faces an uncertain future.

These FDA cases may represent only one to 5 percent of the actual cases that have occurred. Do the math: it equates to at least 242,000 cases of musculoskeletal injury and 40,000 cases of tendon rupture over a period of fifteen years. These numbers are hard to fathom, and a more accurate study should be undertaken.

FREQUENCY OF INJURIES

Different studies have projected different numbers, but one reliable source is the journal *Drug Safety*, which concluded:

> Evidence that exposure to fluoroquinolones is associated with the sudden occurrence of tendinitis is supported by this large population-based study. We can estimate that a single case of rupture of the Achilles tendon would occur for every 5,958 persons treated with fluoroquinolones.

This means there were about 165 cases per million people treated with fluoroquinolones. Since the FDA estimates that in 2011 over 23 million outpatient prescriptions were filled for FQs in the United States, that's 3,795 cases of Achilles ruptures that year.

Onset of Musculoskeletal Injuries

In a 2011 study conducted at the Mayo Clinic, doctors found that "Fluoroquinolone-associated tendinopathy symptoms have occurred as early as two hours after the initial fluoroquinolone exposure and as late as six months after the medication was discontinued."

Could a serious reaction to a FQ occur within hours after the first pill? Yes. I once served as an expert witness in a case of a woman with *myasthenia gravis*, a disease that weakens the muscles, who received Cipro. Her husband was suing the doctor. The woman died within two hours of taking her first Cipro pill. The couple had waited at the doctor's office for fifteen minutes after the woman took Cipro just to be safe, and then they went shopping. As the medication took full effect, it weakened her already compromised respiratory muscles, and she died of asphyxiation before the paramedics could arrive. Even though the Cipro package insert lists myasthenia gravis as a contraindication for using FQs, the doctor had no idea such harm could result. Reading the medical records, I felt that this was a good doctor. If he was unfamiliar with the clear warnings about the serious risks of FQs for his patient, how many other doctors are unfamiliar with this and other contraindications to using FQs?

Other studies have estimated that around two cases of tendon injuries occur per 10,000 people taking a FQ. And with tendon ruptures at about one per 10,000, this translates to about 4,600 tendon injuries and 2,300 tendon ruptures in 2011. These numbers are consistent and therefore credible.

The numbers increase if we consider the unknown yet substantial numbers of inpatient prescriptions for FQs given in United States hospitals. People over sixty have a higher risk of FQ reactions, and people in hospitals are often over sixty. And remember, cases reported to the FDA represent only one to 5 percent of actual incidents, so we need to multiply the above numbers by a factor of as much as twenty or more.

People ask me if there is any difference among FQs in their impact on tendons. A study by the FDA showed the greatest increase in the number of reports of tendon ruptures occurred with Levaquin, a 51 percent increase in new reports of tendon ruptures between 2005 and 2011. Although Cipro had been the most frequently prescribed FQ, numbers of reports of tendon rupture have been consistently higher regarding Levaquin.

Mayo Clinic's Guidelines for Musculoskeletal FTS

In 2011, the Mayo Clinic Sports Medicine Center published their important article, "Musculoskeletal Complications of Fluoroquinolones: Guidelines and Precautions for Usage in the Athletic Population." This groundbreaking article not only provided in-depth information about how FQs injure various tissues on the body, but also provided a stamp of medical legitimacy to musculoskeletal FTS. In this way, the report provides credibility to the fact that FTS is real and should be acknowledged by doctors. The article ends with a list of seven guidelines aimed especially towards athletes and people who participate in regular sports and exercise. The report can also be reasonably applied to all people with injuries from FTS. Here are their guidelines:

1. ***Athletes should avoid all use of fluoroquinolone antibiotics unless no alternative is available.***

    Not only do I subscribe to this recommendation, I think it should apply to everyone of every age. FQs are powerful antibiotics with serious, sometimes permanent side effects. FQs should be reserved for people with serious infections and used only when other, safer antibiotics are not effective. Because I have served as an expert witness in lawsuits in which FQs have done serious harm and doctors have gotten away with gross negligence, I have reservations about whether the system can help people with FTS.

2. ***If an FQ antibiotic is prescribed, the athlete, and ideally the coaching and athletic training staff [and the prescribing doctor] should be made aware of the increased risk for the development of musculoskeletal complications.***

    All patients prescribed FQs should be informed of the FDA-mandated warnings about these drugs' proven potential for severe, disabling injuries. Most people were never given warnings by their doctors and some were not given warnings at their pharmacy.

3. ***Oral or injectable corticosteroids should not be administrated concomitantly with fluoroquinolones.***

    You would think this would be common knowledge among physicians by now, but my experience is that many doctors prescribe steroids at the same time as FQs, and instead identify the condition as autoimmune or rheumatologic or neurologic. My view is that steroids should not be administered simultaneously with FQs unless absolutely necessary, and never within six months after FQ therapy. This includes oral as well as intravenous FQs. There are other options besides FQs.

4. Consideration should be given to supplementation with magnesium and/or antioxidants during the fluoroquinolone treatment course if no contraindications are present.

This is a long overdue recommendation. Mayo Clinic is the first to recommend it. Magnesium is a key element of human physiology, yet most doctors are so adverse to alternative remedies that they scoff at this suggestion. They have no clue that magnesium is vital for treating heart arrhythmias, migraines, Raynaud's disease, palpitations, and high blood pressure. At the same time, it is important to remember that magnesium and other minerals can bind with FQs and impair their absorption and effectiveness in the human body. Therefore, taking a FQ and magnesium or other minerals should be done at least four to six hours apart.

5. Training alterations should begin at the time of the first dose . . . and reductions [in an exercise regimen] should remain throughout the duration of the antibiotic course.

If the athlete shows no symptoms after completing the full course of the FQ, then he can begin to gradually return to full activity, with close monitoring for the development of musculoskeletal or other symptoms.

6. All athletic activity should cease at the onset of symptoms [of FTS], with graduated return to activities when the person is asymptomatic. The fluoroquinolone should be discontinued if possible, and alternative antibiotic treatment should be prescribed if clinically indicated.

7. Close monitoring should continue for one month from conclusion of the [FQ] antibiotic course. The athlete should understand that the symptoms have been reported as late as six months after fluoroquinolone exposure, and prompt medical evaluation should be sought if symptoms develop.

The Mayo Clinic Sports Medicine Center concluded, for emphasis:

Fluoroquinolone antibiotics are associated with a wide array of musculoskeletal complications involving tendon, cartilage, bone, and muscle that are likely under-recognized and under-reported. The pathology of these complications continues to be investigated but appears to be related to alterations in cell-signaling proteins, *as well as direct toxic effects.*

IMPACT ON TENDONS

FQs can cause injury in a single tendon or in many at one time. The main symptom is pain. The tendon injuries caused by FQs resemble overuse injuries in athletes, similar to repetitive stress injuries. Technically, tendons injured by FQs develop abnormal tendon fiber structure, areas of abnormal fibrous tissue, thickening of tendons, and swelling. Studies of FQs in dogs demonstrate reductions in normal collagen and elastin in tendon tissue and reduced production of new collagen, all of which are necessary for healing. Premature cell death (apoptosis) also occurs, which explains the prolonged weakness and slow pace or lack of healing seen in tendon injuries caused by FQs.

Physical Therapy Guidelines

The Mayo Clinic invokes the "T" word, *toxic*, to describe how FQs actually cause harm, sometimes irreversibly, to human tissue. The Mayo Clinic doctors do advise that activity with tendons, cartilage, and joints injured by FQs should be limited as much as possible. Fortunately, FQ injuries often heal within a few weeks or months, but others heal more slowly. We know that healing is hindered in tissues with low metabolic rates such as tendons or cartilage, or in people with limited circulation, as often seen in the elderly.

Renewed activity should be undertaken very gradually, even when pain, swelling, and other symptoms have diminished. Studies in animals show that the abnormal structural changes in tendons from FQs may persist for six months or more, so activity should be undertaken cautiously. In severe cases, the test is that usually most helpful is the MRI. MRIs may or may not show painful tendinitis, but significant tendon tears and ruptures are usually visible. Another method, diagnostic ultrasonography, can sometimes be helpful in assessing tendon injuries.

Physical therapy should be very gentle. Stretching and straining should be avoided. Areas of tightness or spasm can be helped by repeated gentle massage, but if this produces pain, it should be discontinued. Several studies demonstrate protective effects of antioxidants for FQ toxicity, but much more study is needed.

This case was reported in the 2006 journal, *Physical Therapy:*

IMPACT ON CARTILAGE AND BONES

In 2008, the FDA acknowledged in its upgraded warnings on FQs that "Fluoroquinolones exert a toxic effect not only on tendons but also on cartilage, bone and muscle." Several studies have identified the toxic effect of FQs on cartilage. Cartilage lesions display swelling of cartilage matrix, reduced cartilage cell growth and cell metabolism, increased inflammation, and oxidative damage. The Mayo Clinic has also shown that FQs can slow bone healing. Because of this, they recommend avoidance of FQs in patients with fractures or recovering from joint replacement surgery unless FQs are the only effective antibiotic for an infection.

The patient was a forty-one-year-old man, who developed bilateral Achilles tendon pain on the third day of Levaquin use. The physical therapy intervention consisted of an initial phase to reduce stress on the tendon through the use of crutches and orthoses [an external device to modify the structural characteristics of the neuromuscular system], and a second phase to progressively stress the tendon through exercise and functional activities. After eleven weeks of physical therapy (fourteen treatments), the patient's pain decreased from 3/10 to 1/10 on a visual analog scale. His Lower Extremity Functional Scale score increased from 28/80 to 71/80. An overlapping two-phased intervention approach based on connective tissue remodeling principles may be effective in elimination of pain and restoration of function following fluoroquinolone-induced Achilles tendinopathy.

More studies are required to determine the best physical therapy approaches for people with tendon injuries from FQs. If you go to a physical therapist, chiropractor, or anyone who will manipulate your body, make sure the person understands FTS. Make sure he or she has treated other people who have suffered from adverse effects of FQs or similar types of injuries. If possible, bring a copy of the Hall/Mayo Clinic article mentioned above for the therapist to read. Or bring other materials cited in this chapter, or other articles or website materials you have read elsewhere. Working with a physical therapist on your damage from FTS will be a conjoint effort, and it will take time to gradually discover what works best for your body.

IMPACT ON JOINTS

The PDR states that joint pain occurs in approximately one percent of patients. Other studies have reported substantially higher rates. A frequent complaint of people with FQ reactions in a clicking or grating sound from one or more multiple joints with movement. These sounds may occur with or without pain. It is thought that the sounds are the result of swelling or inflammation within the joint, causing audible noise when swollen or inflamed tissues move against one another or against bone.

IMPACT ON MUSCLES

Myalgia, or muscle pain, is a common complaint with FQs. The myalgia may range from mild muscle pain that fades within a few weeks after discontinuing the FQ to severe *myopathy*, or muscle disease. Damaged muscle tissue may also leak the enzyme creatine phosphokinase (CPK) into the bloodstream, resulting in harmful conditions, including a rare, life-threatening muscle breakdown syndrome known as *rhabdomyolysis*. If this is suspected, a blood test for the presence of CPK should be done as soon as possible.

CONCLUSION

Finally in 2008, twenty years after the approval of Cipro, the FDA required stronger warnings in the information on FQs in the PDR and in the package inserts available at pharmacies. The black-box warning, framed by thick black lines, states, "Fluoroquinolones are associated with an increased risk of tendinitis and tendon rupture in all ages." Further down, the warning describes the ravages caused by FQs during animal research:

> In immature rats and dogs, the oral and intravenous administration of FQs resulted in increased osteochondrosis [cartilage damage]. Histo-pathological examination of the weight-bearing joints of immature dogs dosed with fluoroquinolones revealed persistent lesions of the cartilage.

Clearly, the injuries to tendons, muscles, joints and bones from FQs were apparent early on in animal studies and also in the early use of FQs in other countries. Many of the problems we've been seeing for nearly thirty years in the United States certainly could have been avoided or at least minimized. So, too, could many of the other toxicities that FQs can cause people.

3

Toxicity in Central and Peripheral Nervous Systems

The nervous system is comprised of two components: the *peripheral nervous system*, or PNS, and the *central nervous system*, or CNS. The central nervous system is made up of the brain and spinal cord, while the peripheral nervous system comprises sensory and motor nerves to the body from the neck down. The PNS functions to connect the CNS the limbs and organs, relaying messages from the brain and spinal cord to the rest of the body. This is essentially how your body creates movement and perceives the senses. Fluoroquinolones pose a significant danger to the nervous systems.

The initial reports of neurological side effects from FQs came from France in 1982, then Sweden in 1988, and Britain in 1992. The wakeup call about the seriousness of the peripheral nerve damage from FQs came from the Swedish Adverse Drug Reactions Advisory Committee in 1996. The report described thirty-seven cases of peripheral nerve injuries (neuropathies) occurring between 1987 and 1993. Symptoms included abnormal sensations such as tingling or burning (paresthesias), numbness, weakness, loss of sensation, or pain affecting localizing or broad areas of the body. These injuries occurred as early as one hour after taking an FQ to as long as four months later. Most patients recovered after two weeks, but symptoms persisted much longer in others.

PERIPHERAL NEUROPATHIES

Injuries to the peripheral nervous system are known as *peripheral neuropathies*, and can create an array of issues, including numbness in hands and feet, impaired movement, and weakened gland or organ function. In 2001, I reported forty-five cases of serious peripheral neuropathies with FQs. In

33

my survey, 80 percent of the people defined their reactions as severe, with 71 percent lasting more than three months and 58 percent more than a year. The majority of people were young with an average age of forty-two. Prior to FQ treatment, the majority had no previous medical problems.

These are startling numbers in a generally healthy and young population, and the severity and duration of the injuries confirmed that these were not typical side effects. They were toxic reactions, direct injuries to human tissue caused by FQs. In many of these cases, the injuries went beyond the person's nervous system.

Here are some examples:

■ Female, age thirty-nine, given Cipro 500 mg twice daily for ten days. Peripheral neuropathies began after four days but were not recognized by her doctors, so the treatment continued, and then was changed to Levaquin for another fourteen days.

Symptoms: Numbness, increased skin sensitivity, pain on touch, electrical sensations, acute burning sensation all over body, tremors, twitching, disorientation, agitation, racing heart, stomach pain, rashes, visual impairment, temperature intolerance.

Duration: Several years.

Severity: Severe and disabling. Nerve conduction studies abnormal. No prior medical problems.

Subsequent treatment: Steroids worsened symptoms, other medications unhelpful.

■ Male, age thirty-four, received Levaquin 500 mg daily for three weeks for possible prostatitis.

Symptoms: Mild joint pain and visual problems, resolved quickly. Later Levaquin treatment for sinusitis with other symptoms: twitching, numbness, muscle weakness, reduced coordination, shaking, extreme sensitivity to heat and cold, pain in joints of hands, feet, neck and jaw, heart palpitations, severe insomnia and fatigue, extreme nervousness, paranoia, occasional suicidal thoughts, blurred vision in right eye. After four months, some side effects improved but some persisted including palpitations, nervousness, joint pain, neck and jaw pain, visual problems.

Treatment: Valium reduced twitching and partially reduced nervousness and palpitations.

■ Female, age thirty-one, treated with Levaquin 500 mg daily for seven days for sinusitis.

Symptoms: Tingling in both arms initially, then in cheek, then left side of body, which then disappeared. Soon began having burning, numbness, pins and needles, twitching, hypersensitivity, cold intolerance, tendon problems in elbows and wrists with constant pain.

Degree: Severe.

Onset: Two to three days, but "the doctors did not believe I was having an adverse reaction." Ability to work "markedly reduced, had to give up exercise." Minimal improvement over six months, then slight improvement. No previous medical problems.

Fortunately, symptoms of FQ-induced neuropathies are often mild and disappear within weeks or months. On the other hand, severe reactions are not rare. From the third quarter of 1997 through the third quarter of 2012, a span of fifteen years, the FDA received 12,053 reported cases of neurological adverse effects linked to FQs. Our search included only cases in which FQs were the probable cause. Of these cases, 1,585 were defined as "disabling." Remember, only one to 5 percent of adverse reactions get reported to the FDA, so the actual numbers may possibly be hundreds of thousands of cases of peripheral neuropathies from FQs.

A Toxic Combination

Flagyl (metronidazole) is an antibiotic often prescribed for internal infections of the stomach or intestines. It is often combined with a FQ for treating *diverticulitis,* a dangerous and potentially lethal infection of the lower bowel. The combination of these two drugs sometimes works well, but may significantly heighten the risk of peripheral neuropathies. I have received three reports of serious neuropathies from people prescribed Flagyl and a FQ at the same time. Sometimes, combination therapy like this is necessary, but the risk should be acknowledged and the simultaneous use of Flagyl and a FQ should be absolutely avoided when possible.

FDA ACTIONS

Because of the increasing number of reports of neurological injuries with FQs, the FDA contacted experts, including me, in 2004. The FDA officer asked me, "Do you think the cases in your study and other reports are credible?"

"Yes," I replied, "I think the problem is real and serious."

I assume the FDA official was told the same thing by other doctors, because soon thereafter the FDA released an enhanced warning. Nevertheless, the number of reports continued to accelerate. Finally in 2013, after nine more years, the FDA released a new warning about peripheral neuropathies caused by FQs:

> If a patient develops symptoms of peripheral neuropathy, the fluoroquinolone should be stopped, and the patient should be switched to another, non-fluoroquinolone antibacterial drug, unless the benefit of continued treatment with a fluoroquinolone outweighs the risk. Peripheral neuropathy is a nerve disorder occurring in the arms or legs. Symptoms include pain, burning, tingling, numbness, weakness, or a change in sensation to light touch, pain or temperature, or the sense of body position. It can occur at any time during treatment with fluoroquinolones and can last for months to years after the drug is stopped, or may be permanent. Patients using fluoroquinolones who develop any symptoms of peripheral neuropathy should tell their healthcare professionals right away.

And then the FDA finally admitted:

> If you are taking a fluoroquinolone drug, know that it may cause symptoms in the arms or legs such as pain, burning, tingling, numbness, weakness, or a change in sensation to light touch, pain or temperature. These symptoms can occur early in treatment and may be *permanent.*

I can imagine the heated debate at the FDA meeting with medical experts and drug company representatives about whether to include the word "permanent" in this FDA warning for FQs. A word like this can have powerful consequences in legal proceedings about responsibility for FTS events. This one word might empower tens of thousands of people severely injured by FQs to finally earn recognition and, hopefully, fair compensation.

Central Nervous System Toxicities

Current FDA warnings of central nervous system reactions to FQs include the following:

Convulsions, toxic psychoses, increased intracranial pressure, CNS stimulation that may lead to tremors, restlessness, dizziness, lightheadedness, anxiety, phobia, depersonalization, drowsiness, weakness, unsteady walking, confusion, malaise, anorexia, seizures, hallucinations, irritability, paranoia, depression, nightmares, insomnia, and, rarely, suicidal thoughts or acts.

These reactions may occur as early as the first dose. Seizures, which have been linked with Cipro, Levaquin, and other FQs as far back as the 1980s, are a particular concern. The FDA cautions doctors about using FQs in people with a history of seizures or who are taking medications that may predispose them to seizures. FQs lower the seizure threshold in the brain, thereby increasing the risk. If taken with other drugs that can lower the threshold, such as anti-inflammatory medications (NSAIDs), the risk of a seizure with FQs doubles.

To be clear, seizures with FQs can occur in people who do not have these other risk factors, but it is rare. If FQs were needed for a dangerous, life-threatening infection, and there was no alternative antibiotic, the doctor might consider putting the patient on anti-seizure medication.

A "MILD" CASE OF PERIPHERAL NEUROPATHY

I spoke to Linda in mid-March 2014, and she consented to my using her abridged story. My comments are enclosed in the brackets.

I am a thirty-seven-year-old professional woman with two small children who was very healthy until January 2014. I previously did cardio five times a week, weight training three times a week, and ate a healthy diet. On December 27, 2013, I went to Urgent Care for a possible urinary infection and was prescribed Cipro 500 mg twice daily for six days [recommended dosage by the manufacturer is 250 mg twice daily—Linda's dosage was double.]

12/31/2013—Began Cipro prescription for six days, no side effects.

1/5/2014—Finished Cipro prescription, still no side effects.

1/17—First onset: tingling and numbness in both feet.

1/20—Tingling and numbness spread up my calves and elbows.

1/24—Electrical shocks throughout my body. Vertical shocks down my arm or leg. My primary doctor was on vacation, so I met with another physician who diagnosed me with hyperventilation and offered a prescription for Xanax. I declined.

1/27—Tingling and numbness everywhere; deep muscle pain in right arm. Blood tests taken at ER were normal. Referred to neurologist who checked my reflexes and stated that I didn't have MS. He ordered an MRI of my spine and put me on magnesium oxide and methocarbamol [a muscle relaxant.]

1/28–2/11—Continued muscle pains throughout body. One day it would be in my right arm intensely for three hours and disappear, then in left calf, then lower back. Each day it was in a different area and would come and go for a few hours, then a few days with no symptoms.

2/1—Electrical shocks became electrical bursts, feeling like being pinched or stung. Experiencing these thirty to fifty times a day.

2/3—Severe lower back pain.

2/11—Intense pain in right leg, extending from foot to hip and buttocks. While driving, my foot was too weak to hold the brake pedal down, so I had to use both feet to brake [motor nerve neuropathy causing weakness.]

2/12—Muscle pain continuing in right leg from knee to my hip and buttocks. Increased right knee and hip pain with walking. Lower back pain intermittently. Muscle pain has settled in my right leg. Electrical bursts, tingling, and numbness about 80 percent of each day.

2/13—I stopped the muscle relaxers and magnesium oxide because of no benefit [magnesium was a good idea, but magnesium oxide is poorly absorbed by the body.]

2/17—Blood tests for autoimmune disorders normal.

2/20—Saw neurologist: MRIs normal. Neurologist gave me a diagnosis of paresthesia [abnormal nerve symptoms] from no known cause. I didn't understand why I had paresthesia when I was completely healthy before this. I started doing my own research. It was then that I learned about Cipro and realized my symptoms were all similar to the FDA warnings. Note, I told all of my doctors that I'd had a possible urinary tract infection and received Cipro at Urgent Care.

3/6—I asked my primary care physician about Cipro. Seemed like she didn't want to talk about it, so she referred me to these doctors: orthopedist for my hip, rheumatology, endocrinology, another neurologist, cardiologist, urologist, and allergist!

3/10—I met with a second neurologist. He basically told me to get on with my life. When I mentioned Cipro to him, his words were that I needed to stop reading. He ordered an EMG that I will have next week. He indicated that if the EMG came back normal and showed that I didn't have a peripheral neuropathy, then I had to drop the idea of Cipro. I felt very frustrated and angry. [EMG stands for electromyography. It is a nerve test that measures major nerve trunks but often not the small nerves of skin involved in a FQ-caused neuropathy. Either the neurologist was uninformed or ordered the test to shut Linda up.]

3/11—I met with a naturopathic doctor. I told her about my symptoms and then mentioned I had taken Cipro. She was the first doctor who, when I said "Cipro," told me there is a connection with Cipro and nerve problems. [Any doctor can easily see the connection in any official FDA information about FQs, where the warnings are apparent.]

Linda began treatment with the naturopath, receiving intravenous glutathione, which helps some people but not others injured by FQs. Linda's story is typical of the neurological reactions people can encounter with FQs. The failure of Linda's own doctors to identify her reaction and their absurd refusal to consider the possibility of FTS is commonplace. Is it ignorance, fear of lawsuits, or distrust of their own patients' intelligence? Whatever it is, it can be pernicious.

Linda asked me if Cipro was possible cause for the symptoms she was experiencing. I told her, "almost certainly."

"Is there any test that can be done to confirm that?"

"Unfortunately not," I answered.

Linda then asked, "What are the chances of recovering from this? Are there any treatments that might help me?"

I answer questions like these much better than I used to. Because of my experience and increased knowledge, I can comfortably say to people like Linda, "Based on the details of your case, I think your chances are fairly good, even though after three and a half months you still have considerable discomfort, substantial neurological sensory symptoms, and some muscle weakness. On the good side, your symptoms have settled into specific areas, involving no new areas recently. Thus, the toxic reaction seems to have plateaued."

I added, "those are good signs." I told her about both natural and medicinal therapies that might help reduce her symptoms and expedite healing. "We even have a few studies that have shown improvement, not in people, but in animals. It is a start."

Also of note, the doctor had prescribed for Linda 500 mg to be taken twice daily, double the dosage recommended by the manufacturer of Cipro and the FDA for mild urinary tract infections. By doubling Linda's dose of Cipro, the doctor likely increased Linda's risk of adverse effects. The amounts may sound tiny—250 mg versus 500 mg—but medications are some of the most powerful substances in the world. Just look at what one pill can do to some people's systems. Slight increases in dosage may have profound effects. At the proper dose, Linda may not have experienced any side effects, or at least her reaction might have been milder.

CONCLUSION

The overmedication of FQs happens frequently, sometimes with dire consequences. Injuries to the nervous system are no exception. Peripheral neuropathies are debilitating conditions that can negatively impact a person's way of life, as we saw in Linda's case. This cannot go on. Doctors must stop prescribing FQs to patients with mild infections who would have been better off with a safer, milder drug.

4

Toxicity in the Brain, Heart, and Gut

When any antibiotic enters your bloodstream, it travels throughout your body, attacking and killing bacteria as it goes. Fluoroquinolone toxicity syndrome is a pervasive condition that negatively impacts nearly every part of the body. As FQs traverse your body through your blood, they can injure your heart, your digestive system, your mental health, and even your skin, as you will read about in the forthcoming chapter.

CLOSTRIDIUM DIFFICILE

The human intestines contain trillions of friendly bacteria that, in a mutualistic fashion, perform many helpful functions for their human hosts. Located in the intestines, these flora are comprised of many different species. Some people's colons have a minor member of intestinal flora, a bacterium known as *Clostridium difficile,* or C. diff, which is also found in the air, water, soil, and feces. Competition with other bacteria for space and nutrients keeps C. diff under control, so its presence in human intestines isn't typically problematic. Under normal circumstances, people with C. diff in their colons rarely experience adverse symptoms.

However, antibiotics are designed to kill bacteria, and although they are meant to kill a bacterial infection somewhere in the human body, many times they can also kill off large numbers of the natural bacteria lining the intestines. In some cases, the antibiotic destroys the huge numbers of friendly bacteria that keep C. diff in check. The imbalance of intestinal bacteria allows C. diff to proliferate, or grow rapidly out of control.

Minor cases of C. diff overgrowth often results in mild diarrhea. Such brief, mild occurrences may not require treatment. This is why

41

many people receiving antibiotics also take probiotics, healthy bacteria for replenishing the natural flora of the colon. However, a serious infection can occur when the bacterium begins to leak toxins into the lining of the intestines. C. diff infection can cause symptoms ranging from mild to severe, and ultimately create major intestinal problems, including colitis. In some cases, the infection can lead to death. C. diff overgrowth kills 14,000 people a year in the United States.

Antibiotics are the leading cause of C. diff, and the antibiotics most likely to cause C. diff are fluoroquinolones and one other, clindamycin. C. diff epidemics have been reported in many countries. Because of the high risk of C. diff with FQs and clindamycin, the European Center for Disease Prevention has recommended that the use of these drugs be avoided in everyday medical practice except for life-threatening conditions. Treating C. diff superinfections can be difficult. Symptoms can include chronic diarrhea, malaise, weakness, lethargy, abdominal pain, low-grade fever, dehydration, and a distinctive foul stool odor. Successful treatment can take months.

"The most effective method for preventing C. diff overgrowth is proper antimicrobial [antibiotic] prescribing," states one article on this problem. The antibiotics metronidazole (Flagyl) or vancomycin may be necessary to resolve the condition, but these drugs can have many side effects too. Even with these treatments, recurrence of C. diff is about 20 percent. In severe cases of colitis from C. diff overgrowth, surgical removal of the colon may be necessary. That's how serious this disorder can be. Other types of overgrowths can also occur with FQs. Candida overgrowths can occur in the mouth, intestines, or vaginal area. Although these overgrowth reactions are serious, patients are rarely warned about them.

CARDIAC ARRHYTHMIAS

"Experiments in animals have shown that ciprofloxacin has the potential to induce cardiotoxic effects," a 2012 study reported. This was known by the 1990s. By the early 2000s, it was established that serious cardiac effects from FQs, although rare, also occur in humans.

These cardiac changes involve serious alterations in the heart rhythm, known as prolongation of the QT interval, visible on an electrocardiogram. The slowing of this segment of heart activity can cause lightheadedness or outright fainting, which can lead to accidents such as head injuries. An even more severe cardiac irregularity known as *torsade de pointes* (translated as "twisting of the points," due to its unique appearance on the electrocardiogram) can lead to a fatal heart arrhythmia.

Because of the seriousness of these cardiac changes, the FDA has required this warning on all FQ information in package inserts and the PDR:

> Serious heart rhythm changes (QT prolongation and torsades de pointes): Tell your healthcare provider right away if you have a change in your heartbeat [fast or irregular] or if you faint. Cipro may cause a rare heart problem known as prolongation of the QT interval [on an electrocardiogram]. This condition can cause an abnormal heartbeat and can be very dangerous. Occurs especially in the elderly, those with a family history of QT interval prolongation, people with low blood potassium, or those who take anti-arrhythmic medicines.

These cardiac abnormalities from medications are rare. A study by the World Health Organization determines that between 1983 and 1999, 761 cases of QT prolongation were reported. So too were thirty-four deaths from torsades de pointes.

There are only a few medications that are high risk for causing QT prolongation for torsades de pointes. In the early 1990s, Seldane, the first non-sedating antihistamine and best-selling in the world, was withdrawn due to a score of reports of fainting and death due to these cardiac effects. Today, these drug-induced arrhythmias are rare because of better screening in early research. Among current medications, FQs are far down the list of medications causing these problems. FQs do not even top the list of antibiotics known to cause QT prolongation. The rate of this problem with Cipro is about one per million. Nevertheless, you should inform your doctor right away if your heart starts pounding, skipping, or racing, or if you have a history of heart arrhythmias.

PSYCHIATRIC DISORDERS

FQs can trigger a wide range of psychiatric symptoms, from moderate to severe. Some sufferers of fluoroquinolone toxicity develop persisting depression, anxiety, and PTSD. Many complain of "brain fog," in which their thinking and memory feel fuzzy and sluggish. Concentration is impacted, and work performance may be impaired as well. In some people, the brain fog has lasted months or years. In 2013, C.B., a patient who was prescribed Cipro, explained to me:

> In a nutshell, I had a horrific reaction to the antibiotic Cipro three months ago and continue to experience debilitating insomnia, anxiety, and now depression. I have always been averse to taking any prescription medications but took the Cipro because I had a kidney infection. I reacted to the first dose but kept taking it because I was advised to complete the course.
>
> My reaction was "fight or flight" all day and all night. No sleep at all, uncontrollable anxiety, unable to eat, and a change of personality. My heart rate was 165 per minute, more than double my usual heart rate. I have been given many medications to control the symptoms without much improvement, and I am fearful of becoming dependent on the Valium I am being prescribed. I am in bad shape. I am a practicing attorney but have been disabled by this. I simply cannot function.

With treatment, severe psychological reactions, including psychosis, hallucinations, delusions, and acute manic episodes can resolve, but not always. The pharmacovigilance system in France reported 590 cases of psychiatric reactions to fluoroquinolones over a seventeen-year span. The most frequently reported problems were confusion, hallucinations, agitation, delusions, insomnia, and somnolence, or a constant state of extreme drowsiness. 102 of these people required hospitalization. Fortunately, 80 percent of these people responded favorably to treatment. It is not clear whether these 80 percent returned to their pre-FTS levels of functioning, but 20 percent of cases required prolonged psychiatric hospitalization.

Anxiety and Panic Attacks

Compared to mild psychosis or mania, the anxiety disorders caused by FQs may seem mild, but they aren't. Anxiety is mental pain. It can not only greatly impair quality of life, but cause substantial interference with work or social functioning. Chronic anxiety is as unpleasant and distracting as a continual bad headache. It can often trigger panic attacks, or the sudden unleashing of a full-tilt fight or flight reaction, sheer terror, and the overpowering instinct to flee. Panic attacks are short—usually lasting only about ten minutes—but frightening, often inducing an accelerated heartbeat, mental distress, abdominal and chest pain, and nausea.

Repeated episodes not only feel awful, but can also affect a person's ability to venture out or otherwise carry on a normal life.

Depression

FQ-triggered depression can be equally as serious. Anxiety and depression often go hand-in-hand. Depression manifests itself in many different ways, but is typically categorized by a persistent sad, "empty" mood, feelings of helplessness and hopelessness, and a loss of interest in hobbies and activities. Depression can also cause fatigue, memory and concentration problems, irritability, and changes in appetite and weight. In more severe cases, depression can result in thoughts of death or suicide, and suicide attempts.

Post-Traumatic Stress Disorder

You don't have to go to Iraq or Afghanistan to experience post-traumatic stress disorder. PTSD can occur in people exposed to traumatic events of many types. Rape is one example because it alters a person's life and sense of safety for months or years. PTSD is made all the worse by repetitive thoughts and flashbacks that are difficult to erase from the mind.

Official information on FQs doesn't mention PTSD, yet it certainly occurs with severe or prolonged FTS. In my consultations, many people with severe FTS are shocked over how suddenly their lives have changed. They are in pain, unable to sleep, and filled with fears of never recovering and getting their lives back. FTS is utterly disabling. Thus, it is no surprise that the FDA also lists "suicidal thoughts" as an adverse effect with FQs.

People young or old, living a normal life, do not expect to experience sudden severe pain, tendon ruptures, neurological changes, acute pain syndromes, etc., from a simple antibiotic. Nor can they believe that they were prescribed a toxic drug without any warning, especially for a minor infection. Had they been warned, many would have declined treatment with a FQ. Their sense of betrayal by the medical system compounds their distress. And not to forget, some of these stricken people have been led to suicide.

SUNLIGHT PHOTOSENSITIVITY SYNDROME

Many types of drugs, including FQs, can cause photosensitivity, an oversensitivity and reactivity to sunlight. The result can be severe redness, skin burns, and raised vesicles on the skin. While taking an FQ or any other drugs that can cause photosensitivity, you should minimize prolonged exposure to natural sunlight and use protective clothing and sunblock. Also avoid the intense artificial sunlight exposure than can occur in tanning salons.

INFORM YOURSELF

Many other side effects can occur with FQs. You can view them by searching online for the product information for Cipro, Levaquin, Avelox, or the other FQs. Or you can request the package insert for any of these drugs from your pharmacy. Look under the sections for Contraindications, Warnings, Precautions, and Adverse Reactions. Also read the Information for Patients sections. Remember, this information is not a complete list of possible problems with FQs. Rare adverse effects may never get reported or listed.

5

Do Quinolones Damage Human DNA?

Why are the side effects of FQs sometimes so severe? Why do they cause very severe damage, such as shredding strong tendons or scrambling nerves in the central or peripheral nervous system? Why do some of these adverse effects occur so abruptly with just one pill, or, as the FDA now acknowledges, take months to erupt with severe, sometimes permanent, injury? Why, in some cases, can just one or a few FQ pills produce such harm, yet in other cases it can take months for a large tendon to snap abruptly? And why do so many other people take FQs unscathed?

Experts gradually have begun to realize that the answers to these questions lie in the fact that FQs were designed not simply to kill bacteria, but to do so in such a way that can have major blowback in the organisms harboring the infectious bacteria (i.e., laboratory animals, people). First, of their many chemical effects, FQs act as inhibitors of a chemical group known as *topoisomerase enzymes.* Topoisomerase enzymes are vital for maintaining the structural health of the DNA and mitochondria of cells in many types of life forms, including animals and humans. Chemicals that alter the activity of topoisomerase enzymes can cause cell injury or death.

Fluoroquinolones are synthetic antibiotics developed with the ability to inhibit topisomerase enzyme activity in the DNA of bacteria, thereby destroying bacteria's ability to reproduce and spread. They are given the *bactericidal* designation because they kill bacteria outright. This capability has made FQs highly effective antibiotics. Doctors are always concerned that infections can spread and kill patients. A urine infection can spread into a kidney infection, then to a blood infection, then to death. For these reasons, doctors strive to ensure that the antibiotics they choose are strong and effective. This is why FQs became such popular antibiotics in the 1980s and have remained popular for so long. The term "bactericidal" is appealing to doctors because it implies strength and effectiveness. Unfortunately, while FQs were in development, the downside of their significant impact on the body was not fully recognized. Even today, doctors find it hard to believe the reports of serious reactions to FQs by their own patients, and even the updated black-box warnings posted by the FDA.

Many anticancer drugs are also effective via this same mechanism employed by FQs. By blocking the cancer cells' topoisomerase enzyme activity, the cancer cells' DNA is damaged, preventing them from replicating, thereby blocking their ability to divide and spread. Anticancer drug therapy can be harsh to human cells because of the drugs' impact on human DNA. For example, they injure human hair cells, thus some cancer patients suffer hair loss. Fortunately, the hardship of the anticancer therapy proves worthwhile when the cancer is eradicated and the individual's system recovers. However, in a small percentage of cases, the long-term DNA damage from cancer drugs' topoisomerase enzyme inhibition can persist, and, infrequently, later lead to other cancers.

Although early research studies showed FQ's massive injuries to dogs, rats, and mice, the possibility of long-term impact to human DNA was not examined adequately. Why not? This is a question that has been avoided for more than twenty-five years. Many people with FTS believe there has been a cover-up from the start, but this is not really known. Attention is finally being focused on the effects of FQs. In 2003, the book *Fluoroquinoline Antibiotics* stated flatly, "A number of the clinically useful molecules of fluoroquinolones possess different blends of action against [topoisomerase] enzymes, including human topoisomerase II."

Also in 2003, in the journal *Biochemistry*, authors Bromberg, Burgin, and Osheroff described the mechanisms of quinolones' injurious effects on human DNA. In 2012, Adikwu and Brambaifa published "Ciprofloxacin Cardiotoxicity and Hepatotoxicity in Humans and Animals." In their article, they described how Cipro causes toxicity to the DNA in human liver cells, leading to liver disease.

THE FQ-DNA CONNECTION

Joe King, Ph.D., a university professor of quantitative analysis and analytics, is a brilliant mathematician at Carnegie Mellon Research University, where he consults with top corporations all over the world. Joe was a competitive body builder who won competitions, a concert pianist who also played ragtime music, and a radio talk host. After taking Levaquin and then Cipro, he is happy to be alive and able just to walk a few days a week.

Dr. King is also the first person to prove conclusively, scientifically, that FQs can cause vast damage to human DNA, although he would have preferred not to have been the human guinea pig in this endeavor. Here is his story, as he related it to me:

On New Year's Eve 2009, my father and I went to a local restaurant to have dinner and celebrate the beginning of a new year. Two hours after eating a meal of grilled chicken, I was in the ER bent over with excruciating abdominal pain, chills, and a severe headache. I was diagnosed with salmonella food poisoning, caused by the bleaching of spoiled chicken to kill its odor, an illegal process used by some restaurants here.

The ER doctor started an IV infusion of 750 mg of Levaquin. Within thirty minutes I went into convulsions. The doctor blamed this on the salmonella. I then received Levaquin 1,000 mg a day orally for a total of twenty-eight days, then later Cipro for seven days. With each day, I became progressively more incapacitated. I was in and out of the hospital three to four times per week. The third week I was also given prednisone [a steroid] for the excruciating muscle and tendon pain. Steroids are contraindicated with FQs by the FDA, and the steroid/FQ combination accelerated the muscle and tendon deterioration already underway.

On the third day of this regimen, my Achilles tendon and other tendons began rupturing while I was trying to sleep. A neighbor rushed me to the ER, where they tried to prevent the rupturing by packing my body in ice, lowering my body temperature, and beginning an IV infusion of magnesium. This helped temporarily, but both tendons ruptured seven months later, while I was simply watching television.

Two years later, I was hospitalized for long periods while my doctors searched for answers to my pain, weakness, and many other persistent ailments. All during this time, not one doctor attributed my declining health to FQs. Meanwhile, it was strongly suggested to me that my health complaints were psychosomatic. By the end of 2011, I had lost eighty pounds and my muscle mass had dropped continued deterioration of the nerves in my heart and other areas left me with continuous pain.

In 2012, I developed a collapsed coronary artery, which is frequently fatal, but the doctors somehow found a way to save me. The continued deterioration of the nerves in my heart and other areas left me with continuous pain. In May 2012, while standing in the vet's office with my cat, I went into cardiac shock. It was lights out for me. Rushed to the emergency room, turning blue-gray, I was again brought back from the brink of death by my doctors. My heartbeat exceed 200 beats per minute because the primary nerve that controls heart rate and rhythm had frayed. This was a chronic problem traced back to FQ toxicity. The hospital sent me home and suggested I call hospice. My friends came to the hospital to carry me home to die.

Unable to sleep one night, I saw an attorney's ad on television asking people if they'd had tendon ruptures, muscle pain, heart problems, etc. Immediately I contacted him and finally, for the first time, someone explained why I became so sick and incapacitated. I contacted the toxicologist at the Dade County Medical Examiner's Office, who to my surprise I knew from college, and asked if he could run a DNA-adduct [DNA injury] test for me. He directed me to an FBA-certified toxicology lab, and the director told me to fly two vials of blood to her. She had heard of possible problems with FQs. She did the test as a favor to me and as an important scientific investigation.

The method she used was gas chromatography mass spectrometry, and the DNA was analyzed by the most modern methods. Soon, she informed me that the FQs and some metabolites were found adducted [attached abnormally] to my DNA. Next, she contacted some heavyweights in the fields of pharmaceutical toxicology, and pharmaceutical research and development. She also contacted several medical schools and research across the country, including the University of Utah School of Medicine's Center for Human Poisoning, the leading research center in the world. Thus, we involved the very top toxicology resources anywhere. The unanimous conclusion was that my DNA had been adducted by Levaquin and Cipro. This was the first conclusive proof in the world that FQs truly damaged human DNA.

The experts also had another message for me: the effect of the FQ poisoning was irreversible. Several weeks later, I collapsed in my backyard and was taken to the same ER. The doctors immediately told me, "Why are you back? We told you there is nothing wrong with you." I'd gone there because I could not move my legs or body, but they did not want to listen.

I threw the toxicology report at them and said, "I have been poisoned by Levaquin and Cipro, and I have the toxicology analysis to prove it from an FBI-certified lab. The drug has adducted to my DNA permanently, and you guys are going to figure out right now what to do to fix me. If not, tomorrow you will be talking to my attorney!"

They read the report. The doctors immediately changed the way they dealt with me. I no longer had doubtful doctors who were dismissive, sometimes insulting. From that point on, no doctor could argue with me about whether I'd been poisoned by FQs. I remember vividly a group of emergency doctors yelling at me at the top of their voices, "Mr. King, there is *nothing* wrong with you! Do not come back to this ER and tie it up when we have real sick people waiting to get help!"

About fifteen minutes after I showed them the evidence, the entire medical staff, including the medical director, came into my room and apologized for doubting me and for the way they had spoken to me and treated me. The doctors told me that they had never heard that the FQs could do such damage to human tissue, and they were greatly worried about other patients who manifested similar symptoms. Then they said the most wonderful thing to me: "Mr. King, what can we all do to help you? Just tell us and it will be done."

What happened that day in the emergency room quickly spread throughout the medical community in South Florida, and soon I became known as the Professor of DNA-adducts! Since then I've had more than 100 doctors in South Florida contact me for toxicity information on FQs and several told me in confidence that they have always considered FQs to be dangerous.

Today, the doctors at the ER call me "Humpty Dumpty Man" because I always arrive with multiple problems and they have to try to patch me up together again. Gallows humor is better than no humor, right? Today I have constant pain, frequent tendon ruptures, and erosion of tissue in different areas. There are no pain medications that control the pain. Occasionally, my doctors will infuse two grams of IV magnesium, which takes the edge off the pain for one or two days. Neither anti-inflammatory drugs nor opiates, not even Vicodin, Oxycontin or morphine work anymore. But we are making strides in getting the word out about the dangers of FQs.

I spoke to Dr. King again in June 2014 and February 2015. His medical problems continue, but he sounded good, just as sharp as always, and displayed a good philosophy about his situation. He remains in frequent contact with many others who are afflicted by fluoroquinolone toxicity. In May 2014, a group went to Washington, D.C., some in wheelchairs, to testify in front of a Senate subcommittee finally investigating the FTS tragedy. I was told that the subcommittee was given the letter I had written for the Senate committee, which is placed at the beginning of this book. The subcommittee discussed pressuring the FDA to initiate studies to investigate FQs and their method of action. Whether this actually leads to anything productive remains to be seen. Let's hope so.

THE DNA-ADDUCT TESTING PROJECT

Despite the fact that reports of major, extended injuries from FQs in humans dates back thirty years, no in-depth studies have addressed the obvious possibility of genetic damage in humans from FQs. Finally, in late 2013, a team of medical scientists undertook research to examine whether FQs actually could impact human DNA. In spring 2014, a team led by Dr. King released the results of the Fluoroquinolone DNA-Adduct Testing Project.

DNA-adducts are altered forms of DNA that occur from exposure to a toxin or carcinogen. Once a section of healthy DNA becomes adducted, this section of the gene becomes compromised and dysfunctional. The scientific term for this is *genotoxicity*, or toxicity to genes. A DNA-adduct subsequently will block the corresponding gene's expression and ability to replicate correctly. This in turn hinders the gene's ability to correctly direct the protein synthesis necessary for its repair. The result of this genotoxicity may be aberrant proteins and mutated cells. The body may then attack these abnormal cells via an autoimmune reaction causing severe inflammation, pain, weakness, fatigue, and failure to heal. This study established beyond a doubt that FQs can cause genotoxicity.

The team undertaking this study included a biochemist, microbiologist, pharmacologist, toxicologist, and biogenetic engineer. Beginning the study in 2013, the researchers selected five people at random who had developed severe chronic conditions in close association with FQ use. All had been in good health, physically active, gainfully employed, and with no preexisting medical conditions prior to being prescribed FQs in 2009 or 2010. [*See* Table 7.1.]

The study results: Samples from all five subjects with FTS showed multiple markers of DNA-adducts in their cellular and mitochondrial DNA. The list of specific DNA-adducts is long and technical, but the findings overall were grossly abnormal. On the other hand, two subjects recruited for the placebo group with no history of taking FQs and no medical problems displayed no markers of genetic adducts. The conclusion was unequivocal: the genetic abnormalities found in the study group

TABLE 7.1. FLUOROQUINOLONE DNA-ADDUCT TESTING PROJECT				
Subject	Age	Occupation	Antibiotic	Duration
Female	51	Professional	Cipro, Levaquin	30 days
Female	38	Professional	Levaquin	1 day
Female	42	Consultant	Cipro	7 days
Male	47	Professional	Cipro	42 days
Male	47	Professional	Levaquin	7 days

were undeniable, and the FQs were the only profitable explanation for these people's severe, prolonged illnesses.

Dr. King made an urgent plea: "Doctors must understand that a patient with FTS is not having a simple adverse reaction. The patient's original genetic profile has been altered, mutated, and their symptoms and health complaints are real, not psychosomatic. The doctor's evaluation can easily begin by simply asking whether the patient had been prescribed a FQ antibiotic."

It is also important to note that the average age of the subjects in the study was forty-five years. Many doctors believe that FTS only occurs in people above age sixty. With this inaccurate perception, they often dismiss younger patients badly injured by FQs. It is important to broaden their understanding of FTS so they can help those in need.

Dr. King also poses the following disturbing questions: "Has a monster been created? Has this class of antibiotics created a long-term genotoxicity with future generational problems? Can our exponential upswing of neurological, musculoskeletal, and phantom health problems be associated with these antibiotics' use? Today, this is highly suspected. Current data, research, and results are pointing an accusing finger at the fluoroquinolones."

CONCLUSION

In summary, can FQs injure human DNA? The answer seems, undeniably, "Yes." This has long been seen in bacteria and several types of laboratory animals. The biochemical mechanisms of FQs' unique destructiveness in both the mitochondria and the nuclei of cells is known to occur via at least two methods: adduction to the DNA and topoisomerase II activity. Now we know that these damaging actions have occurred not only in other species, but also via the study described above in humans. And if we include the tens of thousands of reports to the FDA of FTS, many thousands more Americans have been injured genetically.

Although there have been many well-known medication disasters in history, there has never been a medication disaster equaling this. The essential question is now twofold: Can serious FQ reactions be prevented? And can people injured by FQs be helped? I will discuss these two key questions in Part 2, The Solution.

PART TWO

The Solution

6

The Benefits of Magnesium

There is a surprising amount of evidence about probable causes and possible therapies for fluoroquinolone toxicity syndrome. Toxicities have been reported with FQs since the 1980s. Today, the medical literature continues to report cases of injuries, many serious and lasting so long that the FDA acknowledges some FQ-generated damage is permanent.

Nonetheless, many doctors, relaying what drug reps tell them, tell their patients that FQs are safe and have only a few mild, brief side effects. Yet, after suffering from these toxic effects and not healing, many patients find themselves making the rounds of rheumatologists, neurologists, orthopedists, etc., and often receive nothing but disagreement, disbelief, and dismissal. Alternative doctors have been more supportive overall, yet similarly helpless to provide assistance.

Dr. Joe King provided a breakthrough in spring 2014 with his scientific study proving that people with fluoroquinolone toxicity syndrome display DNA abnormalities in the cells of injured tissues. This explains the pain and long duration of FQ injuries and why healing is slow or absent. That the FDA acknowledges some effects of FTS as permanent means they don't understand it well enough to suggest how to fix the problem.

Finally, we may be getting closer to understanding FTS and perhaps scaling back the vast number of incidents. This would be a great breakthrough since an estimated 30 million people receive FQs annually in the United States. The FDA has received nearly 50,000 reports of serious FTS, yet, by its own studies, it usually hears about only one to 5 percent of all side effect cases. So we suspect that the actual number of FTS cases a year is vastly more than the FDA acknowledges.

As you read in the introduction to this book, when the CDC was recommending Cipro to everyone during the anthrax scare fifteen years ago, I reported forty-five cases of severe FTS in the article "Peripheral Neuropathy Associated with Fluoroquinolone Antibiotics." Now, finally, we have a few answers and substantial evidence that magnesium plays an important role in treating the symptoms of FQ toxicity.

STUDIES ON MAGNESIUM AND TOXICITY

Animal studies between 1995 and 2002 indicate that higher numbers of joint and cartilage injuries were caused when feeding FQs to animals. These studies demonstrated that FQs *chelate*, or bind, magnesium, inactivating it in a way that induces magnesium deficiency within the animals' cells. The FQs cause tissue damage and magnesium deficiency at the same time, thereby promoting further tissue injury. The result is damage more severe than caused by the FQ itself. You don't have to read every word of these abstracts to get the picture. If you obtain the full articles, they spell it out even more clearly.

The publication of the following nine key magnesium studies should have sounded alarm bells:

Year: 1995

Journal: *Antimicrobial Agents and Chemotherapy*

Findings: "Magnesium deficiency induces joint cartilage lesions in juvenile rats which are identical to quinolone-induced arthropathies (abnormalities)." Quinolones accumulate in cartilage and form chelate complexes that can inactivate substances with magnesium. They possess the potential to induce a deficiency of active magnesium. Cartilage abnormalities were found in the knee joints of rats that were placed on magnesium-deficient diets. Deficiency occurred in rats given the FQ ofloxacin, including those with a normal diet. Cartilage injuries in rats treated with ofloxacin plus magnesium deficiency were more pronounced. The authors suggested that if patients must be treated with quinolones for serious infections, it seems wise to ensure that patients do not have a disturbed magnesium balance.

Year: 1996

Journal: *Archives of Toxicology*

My Experience With Magnesium as Doctor and Patient

Magnesium is abundant in the universe, on earth, and in our bodies, yet our doctors are not taught much about it. When I mention magnesium to doctors as a proven therapy for migraines, their eyes glaze over. They think that migraines can only be treated with drugs and that magnesium is a mere mineral, something offered by chiropractors or herbalists who cannot prescribe drugs. Doctors don't understand that there is a physiological mechanism underlying migraines, and that this mechanism is often lacking magnesium, which is needed for normal neurovascular functioning. I learned years ago that 75 percent of Western populations have inadequate levels of magnesium. When I tell migraine patients that they lack magnesium and should tell their doctors, they return and tell me, "My doctor isn't interested."

In 1998, I discovered that magnesium could aid my severe, horribly painful nerve condition, erythromelalgia, which disabled me for a decade. I tried many medications without benefit, yet the disease unexpectedly responded to a long series of intravenous Myers' cocktails, an alternative medical mixture of intravenous vitamins and minerals provided by an integrative doctor. It took a while for us to realize the key ingredient was magnesium. We also found that with multiple daily oral doses of magnesium, my condition gradually stabilized, and eventually I reopened my practice and my life resumed. I learned then that magnesium is a vital factor for normal functioning of the human system, especially the nervous system.

Like most doctors, I always assumed that medical research was the most thorough, and I was shocked when I found that magnesium research outweighed anything I'd ever seen. For example, for Lipitor (atvorvastatin), the top-selling drug in America at the time, there were nearly 7,000 publications listed in the United States Library of Medicine of the National Institutes of Health (PubMed.org). That is a lot of studies, yet compare that to magnesium's 92,776 listings—fifteen times more. Despite the overwhelming literature, general practitioners know little about magnesium and therefore doubt its importance for normal human physiology.

Yet, how can we forget about the everyday use of magnesium in hospital cardiac care units to halt dangerous cardiac arrhythmias? And in maternity care units, where magnesium is given intravenously to blunt a woman's dangerously high blood pressure and reduce her risks of seizures from maternal preeclampsia? Magnesium's importance for normal functioning in humans is not a stretch at all.

During my journey involving magnesium, I was privileged to meet the "queen of magnesium," Mildred Seelig, M.D., a bright and engaging woman. She carried a message that was important for everyone and unexpectedly important for us who have been thrust into the FQ world.

"I was working at a drug company," she told me. "I'd just finished my training and was evaluating a new medication for its antihypertensive qualities. While using magnesium as an inert substance for comparison, I found that it wasn't actually inert at all, but worked better and was overall the more beneficial medication. So I began studying it, which led me on a new career path—to learn and teach about magnesium."

She looked at me and laughed, then said, "You, my young friend, are on a similar path. The mainstream doctors will be suspicious of you because you think differently, but like me, you'll learn a lot that will amaze you."

My own life medicine had already taken several unexpected turns. I began as a general practitioner, then moved to UCLA for research in acupuncture, then to psychiatry at the University of California, San Diego. After many years, I began writing about my real interest: medication side effects and why they perennially are amid the top five causes of death in the United States, behind heart disease, cancer, and strokes. My first article examined the problems and serious omissions of the *Physician's Desk Reference,* the bible of medication information that doctors use to guide them when prescribing drugs. Unaccustomed to writing for medical journals, I asked Paul Insel, M.D., UCSD's chairman of pharmacology, for assistance. I didn't realize that he was the president of the American College of Clinical Pharmacology and Therapeutics. This was and is the top pharmacology association in the United States, and Dr. Insel was knowledgeable and gracious, too. I lucked out.

Several medical journal articles later, the *New York Times* wrote about my work in its science section, cover page, and then *Newsweek* published an article they commissioned from me. Around the same time, a woman named Beth W. contacted me with information about the terrible adverse effects she was experiencing after taking Cipro. Of course I'd heard of Cipro, even took it a couple of times, but I had no idea of its risks. I happened to be taking magnesium at the time I took the Cipro, and this may have protected me.

The timing of my 2001 article on forty-five cases of severe neuropathies caused by FTS was also lucky. Three of the four peer reviewers of the article opposed its publication: "too negative ... too controversial ... insufficiently supported by the data." But I'd done it as a survey, like taking a poll. I'd become savvy enough in my career not to claim proof when I was only trying to raise awareness. As a survey, it served well to merely point out that a serious FQ problem might be happening.

"You were the one who sounded the alarm, who raised our awareness," Dr. King told me recently. I had no idea of the impact. Now I hope to raise more and maybe even offer a way to prevent many cases of FTS.

After a brief stint on NPR in autumn 2001, people began calling my office. One here. One there. Just a trickle. I now estimate I've spoken to 500 people. Most of the callers want to speak to a doctor who will talk straight about FQs. These people are sick medically, and they know it. Yet most doctors continue to insist the drugs are safe and these people are misguided. Knowing that these people have gotten some of their information from the internet (as if that's a sin), the doctors ask, how accurate could it be? Many doctors even refuse to look at the black-box warnings written by the drug companies under FDA direction. I've never understood how doctors can reject this type of information. We've seen medical catastrophes before. And now we have another.

Findings: This group also saw ofloxacin-induced cartilage defects, likely due to chelation of magnesium, thus causing a functional deficit of available magnesium in joint cartilage.

Year: 1997

Journal: *Archives of Toxicology*

Findings: This article says that FQs are known for their ability to form chelate complexes with magnesium. Cartilage lesions seen in young animals after FQ treatment probably were due to lack of functionally available magnesium. This study measured the distribution of magnesium, calcium, and ofloxacin in cartilage. During FQ toxicity, magnesium in juvenile cartilage was very low. FQ may have lowered the concentration of functionally available magnesium below a critical level.

Year: 1998

Journal: *Scanning*

Findings: FQs have been shown to provide benefit for children with chronic pulmonary disease, as with cystic fibrosis. Yet FQs have been seen to cause cartilage injury in experimental animals. This study examined cartilage cells of hip joints of young rats, showing that FQs were related to abnormalities seen in cell shape, structure and activity.

Year: 1999

Journal: *Drugs*

Findings: FQs associated with adverse effects such as cartilage abnormality "can probably be explained by the magnesium-chelating properties of these drugs." These tendon injuries can occur very late, as late as many months after treatment. "Overall, quinolones are well tolerated drugs ... but their specific toxic potentials have to be considered" when used for treating bacterial infections.

Year: 2000

Journal: *Antimicrobial Agents and Chemotherapy*

Findings: This study performed extensive electron microscopic examinations of Achilles tendon specimens from rats treated with ofloxacin. Three days after treatment, the Achilles tendon cells displayed multiple abnormalities. There were degenerative alterations in the cytoplasm due to swelling of cell organelles. Other signs were the appearance of cell debris. The tendon cells of the young rats treated once with ofloxacin underwent examination. The FQ-induced abnormal findings were found in joints and tendons, signs of the same toxic effects.

Year: 2001

Journal: *Archives of Toxicology*

Findings: The title, "Biochemical Changes in Achilles Tendons from Juvenile Dogs After Treatment With Ciprofloxacin or Feeding a Magnesium-Deficient Diet," says it all. After studying the effects of FQs on the Achilles tendons of magnesium-deficient dogs after autopsy, the researchers concluded, "These findings support our hypothesis that quinolone-induced toxic effects on connective tissue structures are due to the magnesium antagonistic effects of these antibacterial agents. They also indicate that patients with a latent magnesium deficiency could be at an increased risk of quinolone-induced tendon disorders."

Year: 2001

Journal: *Annals of Pharmacotherapy*

Findings: Three doses of Levaquin triggered seizures in a seventy-five-year-old woman who was found to have a low level of serum magnesium. One month later, she had another seizure when prescribed Cipro, and was found to have low sodium, indicating kidney failure. Risk factors for FQ-induced seizures include electrolyte imbalances (such as of magnesium or sodium deficiency). Her dosage likely was not adjusted for her kidney failure, or for a history of seizures (which she did not have).

Year: 2002

Journal: *Antimicrobial Agents in Chemotherapy*

Findings: Studies on ofloxacin in young rats showed that magnesium-deficient diets produced significantly lower magnesium levels in bone and plasma, as well as increased in cartilage lesions compared to rats fed normal diets. The researchers found "The incidence of ofloxacin-induced lesions was higher in the magnesium-deficient animals, suggesting a synergistic effect." They recommended caution using FQs or pediatric populations.

These nine studies indicate how FQs worsened the number, severity, and duration of injuries related to magnesium deficiency. The evidence is very consistent. We've long known that FQs directly cause myriad tissue injuries. Many of these, especially many common ones such as musculoskeletal injuries (joints, tendons, muscle, cartilage) can be attributed directly to the effects of FQs. And as the studies above show, we now know that magnesium deficiency can cause similar musculoskeletal injuries. And now we can see clearly that FQs and magnesium deficiency together can create a toxic brew that is even more destructive.

In the first published article in 1995, the researchers agreed that the mechanism in rats and humans was similar. They stated explicitly, "If juvenile patients must be treated with quinolones for serious infections, it seems prudent to ensure that these patients do not have a disturbed magnesium balance." Yes, it would have been prudent, to say the least. This statement was published twenty years ago, and there still hasn't been much effort to heed it. In 2001, the researchers wrote, "Patients with a latent magnesium deficiency could be at an increased risk of quinolone-induced tendon disorders." With these data from eight successive years of published studies, there was little doubt about it. Many types of injuries have increased since FQs were released for public use.

A Pathway to Prevention?

You would think that by 2002, with all the research and information regarding magnesium, medical authorities would have jumped at recommending magnesium therapy for people starting FQ treatment. The evidence was not thin. The nine studies I presented show that FQs bind magnesium and keep it from being utilized properly in the formation and rebuilding of the musculoskeletal and other systems in rats. This evidence is highly relevant because the FQ-related injuries that FQs caused in rats are similar to those seen in humans with FTS.

The risks of FQs were known from the 1970s, but we didn't know why. By 2002, with the publication of these studies, the risks were clear. We now understand that FQs bind magnesium, an element vital for normal physiological functioning and healing. Since this has been repeatedly proven in young rats in 1995 and thereafter, we must ask how many cases of FTS might have been prevented by 2002, if the alarm about FQs' causing magnesium deficiency had been sounded.

It also seems that if the magnesium deficiencies are not rectified, it is unlikely that people's injuries will heal. Recovery likely will be further stalled, perhaps indefinitely. Isn't this what we have been seeing in so many cases of FTS from the beginning? This begs the question: when a person is experiencing severe side effects after using FQs, what are their chances of recovery? Remember, the average person's diet is low in magnesium. About 75 percent of Westerners are deficient in magnesium to begin with. So what are people's chances of healing from fluoroquinolone toxicity with an already low magnesium intake?

The question is, why haven't we—both patients and doctors— been informed about this? At least from 1995 to 2002 when these study results were published and confirmed over and over again, why weren't we told about the role of magnesium and the interplay between it and FQs? This is vital information for doctors and patients alike. Why wasn't a plan of action laid out? Why wasn't something done? Why hasn't anything been done since then or being done now, ten to twenty years later?

A STUDY ON MAGNESIUM AND VITAMIN E

In 2007, a study was published that should have prompted immediate steps toward halting the Cipro catastrophe. This study by Pfister, Mazur, Vormann, and Stahlmann was published in the respected journal *Antimicrobial Agents and Chemotherapy*. The publishers must have understood the study's importance because they pre-published it online on January 8, 2007, rather than wait for the publication in the hard copy of the journal in March. The title itself should have attracted wide interest: "Diminished Cirpofloxacin-Induced Chondrotoxicity by Supplementation with Magnesium and Vitamin E in Immature Rats."

After the studies performed from 1995 to 2002, this research seems the logical next step. The authors of this research explained why:

> Quinolone-induced chondrotoxicity [cartilage damage] in juvenile rats and multiple other species has been demonstrated previously. Identical damages can be induced in immature rats by feeding them a magnesium-deficient diet. The objective of this present study was to investigate whether, in reverse, oral supplementation with magnesium, vitamin E, or both can diminish the typical quinolone-induced arthropathy [joint injuries] in juvenile Wistar rats.

The researchers separated young rats into four groups of twelve rats each. One of the groups received a standard diet, one group received a vitamin E-enriched diet, one group a magnesium-enriched diet, and the fourth group a diet enriched with magnesium plus vitamin E.

Each group received their diets for ten days, but on the eighth day, all of the rats received two doses subcutaneously of 600 mg per kilogram of Cipro. Two days later, the animals were sacrificed. Cartilage samples from their knee joints were examined microscopically for typical quinolone-induced lesions. The concentrations of magnesium and vitamin E in cartilage and plasma were measured and, as expected, were found to be higher in the animals receiving the enriched feeds. In contrast, a statistically significant higher number of cartilage lesions were identified in tissues from the group receiving the standard feed, that is, the standard diet without additional supplementation. Tissue from the groups receiving magnesium or vitamin E both displayed significantly fewer injuries in comparison to the group receiving the standard diet. Remember, all of the rats received the Cipro injections, too. (*See* Table 9.1.)

Group	Percent Reduction of Cartilage Injuries	Number of Lesions
TABLE 9.1. NUMBER & PERCENT REDUCTION OF CARTILAGE INJURIES IN RATS RECEIVING CIPRO		
1, Standard Feed	—	17
2, Vitamin E-Enriched Feed	41	10
3, Magnesium-Enriched Feed	65	6
4, Vitamin E/Magnesium Feed	82	3

The researchers noted that in Group 4, the number of injuries was reduced by 82 percent in comparison to the rats receiving only Cipro and the standard feed in Group 1. So if you were prescribed a FQ, you were treated pretty much like the rats that received the standard feed. This was the group of rats with the greatest extent of FTS injury. In fact, everyone who has been prescribed a FQ has been treated like this group of rats. They received no instructions for the enrichment of vitamin E or magnesium or both that protected the rats. Remember, enriched feeds reduced FQ-related injuries by 41 percent (vitamin E), 65 percent (magnesium), or 82 percent (vitamin E plus magnesium). As far as I know, humans have never been advised to take these supplements to protect themselves while taking a FQ.

THE PRILOSEC-MAGNESIUM EXAMPLE

In March 2011, the FDA notified Americans that the popular drugs known as proton pump inhibitors (PPIs) could cause magnesium deficiency in people who take these drugs for three months or longer. This was an important finding because many people have chronic upper gastrointestinal conditions such as hiatal hernia, ulcers, or diseases of the esophagus that require prolonged stomach acid suppressive therapy with PPIs. Although the package inserts of these medications warn people against taking them for lengthy periods, many people find it necessary to remain on PPIs for years. PPIs including Prilosec, Prevacid, Protonix, Nexium, and others are among our best-selling drugs. The manufacturer of Prilosec is solving the problem by adding magnesium to the formulation of Prilosec itself.

The FDA also warns that having a low magnesium level can be a problem for people who take the heart drug digoxin or who take diuretics for high blood pressure. Diuretics are well-known to wash out potassium, but less well-known for their tendency to deplete magnesium, too. Some of the signs of a low magnesium level may include dizziness, jitteriness, rapid heart rhythm or heartbeat, shaking or tremors, jerking movements, muscle weakness, muscle aches, spasms of the hands or feet, cramps, and seizures. PPIs like Prilosec can cause magnesium deficiency after one year of use, and in some cases as early as three months. Magnesium deficiency is infrequent in people using over-the-counter forms of Prilosec, Nexium, and Prevacid within their manufacturer's guidelines.

We might ask, why haven't the FQs been marketed similarly to Prilosec, with enough magnesium to keep people's cellular levels adequate? Wouldn't this solve the FQs' tendency to bind and inactivate magnesium in our cells? The difficulty of this approach is that magnesium also binds FQs, inactivating FQs' antibacterial activity, the purpose for which FQs were developed. Magnesium could make the drugs useless.

FQs and Magnesium

There may be another approach. Studies have been conducted with FQs and antacids containing minerals such as magnesium. It was found that the minerals can be taken four hours apart from FQs without affecting either's absorption or activity. So why hasn't this approach using FQs and magnesium hours apart been tested by the drug companies and FDA?

Such an approach might be effective. Would it work? It must be remembered that in the 2007 study, magnesium enrichment was indeed effective in reducing the number of FQ injuries by 65 percent, a very impressive number. However, the rats were given feed enriched with magnesium for seven days before they received Cipro on the eighth day. Would a single dosage of magnesium several hours before the first FQ pill make a difference? We don't know, but it might be worth testing. I would certainly advise doctors to tell their patients requiring FQ therapy about this. If not feasible, I might consider providing an intravenous infusion of

An Approach to Magnesium Treatments

After having an emergency appendectomy in early January 2015, Sean, age thirty-three, returned to his doctor twelve days later because of increasing pain and inflammation around the incision site. The doctor prescribed the FQ antibiotic Levaquin, and another anti-infective, Flagyl (metronidazole). Flagyl is often used for infections involving the intestine because of its effectiveness against many gram-negative bacteria. As you previously learned, Flagyl is sometimes used with a FQ because of the very broad range of coverage the two types of drugs provide together.

Sean experienced harsh side effects— not surprising because both drugs are known for these. I've had a few cases reported with this drug combination, and each person reported many adverse effects. Sean reported burning pain in his arms, severe headaches, muscle twitches, feeling unsteady on his feet, confusion, foggy thinking, extreme fatigue, severe anxiety, panic attacks, and loss of appetite. In addition, his temperature was below normal, so on many nights he felt very cold and would sit next to a space heater until he could fall asleep. In addition, he had terrible nightmares with night sweats that drenched his clothing and sheets. That's when he discontinued the antibiotics.

His symptoms continued, with headaches and panic attacks so severe he could barely function. He went to a nearby emergency room, where he was given opiates for his severe headaches. Unimproved, he returned to the ER the next day, where he received a more thorough evaluation including many tests: CT scan, MRI, lumbar puncture, blood and urine tests. Everything was normal except for a low white cell count, a nonspecific finding. They gave him morphine for his headache and sent him home again.

"By the time I saw Sean," his girlfriend told me, "he had developed a deep, throaty cough, and he could do nothing but lie down and stare into space. He was suffering mentally from confusion, depression, and a lot of fear. He also told me that he felt hollow and had 'dark thoughts' and a feeling of overwhelming detachment. At night he would ask me to lie down next to him and hold his hand because he was so afraid. This was not his normal state of being!"

Sean went to another emergency room where he knew the doctor. The doctor was puzzled by his symptoms but gave Sean an IV with magnesium, thinking perhaps he was having a severe migraine with associated physical symptoms. Sean began to feel better. Within an hour, he felt less tense, and his anxiety gradually melted away.

After leaving the ER, Sean continued taking magnesium. He took six pills of magnesium L-threonate each day. At 144 mg per capsule, he was taking 850 mg a day, a strong but not excessive dosage for an acute situation. When I spoke to him three weeks later, he was still struggling with insomnia, but his night sweats had disappeared. Sean was also taking a combination of supplements including pyrroloquinoline quinone (PQQ) for boosting his energy, as well as salmon oil, B complex, zinc, probiotics and flax oil. He was also eating a healthy organic diet that included vitamin-enriched smoothies and avoiding sugar. I am not recommending Sean's combinations of therapies as a specific protocol, but they provide a good example of what people attempt, trying to find things that help. I do believe the magnesium he received was helpful. I asked Sean how he was doing at that point.

"I still need to lie down a lot," he told me. "On the good side, the only medication I need anymore is for sleep. Overall, I'd say I have been improving gradually but steadily." I told him about the other possible therapies for him, including supplements and medications.

This case is the first in which I've heard about the use of intravenous magnesium while an FTS reaction was unfolding. People have tried other infusions such as glutathione, but those reports were mixed at best. Sean's experience was like a double-blind study, since he had no idea what the problem was. He'd never heard of Levaquin or fluoroquinolones or their toxicities. The doctor thought he was treating a severe migraine syndrome. Yet both seem satisfied that improvement had indeed occurred. If we could have a series of ten cases like this, we might finally be able to convince the medical establishment that magnesium can treat FTS.

At the very least, the information presented in this chapter and the previous chapter on magnesium deserves immediate examination. I urge the FDA and drug companies to move forward on this. Medical institutions must also play a role, because they are often the first ones to provide treatment and so far they do not know what to do. Remember Dr. Joe King's experience in a South Florida emergency room? We must find out if magnesium can help us dramatically reduce the occurrence and severity of the fluoroquinolone catastrophe that has been going on for almost thirty years.

magnesium, in which a larger dose of magnesium could be given. In addition, I would also consider magnesium supplementation once or twice every day, four to six hours away from the FQ dosage. This could be easy to do with Levaquin, which can be taking once daily upon arising. The magnesium could be conveniently spaced in between the drug doses.

Working like this with animals and then people, we could perform proper studies that would allow use to see if we could truly reduce the incidence of FTS. This would provide vital data for doctors to use with patients requiring FQs. It would be a welcome change to help doctors work together with their patients to prevent FTS before it happens.

HOW TO TAKE MAGNESIUM FOR FLUOROQUINOLONE TOXICITY SYNDROME (FTS)

"How should I take magnesium?" This is a question I am asked often. As I've shown, there are far more papers in the medical journals on magnesium than on many top-selling drugs. That's because magnesium is one of the most important elements in the body. Studies have shown that magnesium provides benefits not only for hypertension, but also for migraines, Raynaud's phenomenon, and many other conditions of the human neurovascular system. And it is essential for cellular healing.

Types of Magnesium

Some people have a favorite form of magnesium. There are many types: oxide, citrate, orotate, chloride, lactate, sulfate, carbonate, threonate, taurate, and glycinate. Many alternative practitioners favor magnesium chloride. Although I tried it many times, I never found it effective against my neurological disorder. Many other types of magnesium were helpful for me. One of them was magnesium sulfate, the type mainstream doctors use for infusions in hospitals.

Lately, a favorite type of magnesium seems to be glycinate or triglycinate. People have mentioned having fewer side effects with it. Glycinate is what Kerri Knox, R.N., recommends in her writings about natural treatments for FTS. I also recommend magnesium glycinate to people trying to heal their FTS. However, if others prefer another form of magnesium, that's fine with me since the magnesium itself is the key, not the second part of the compound. Different people have different opinions on this. Some types of magnesium come in granules, such as Natural Calm, a popular form of magnesium citrate. You can dissolve this preparation in water, thereby facilitating its absorption. Another common form is the dissolvable magnesium sulfate in Epsom salts for baths. The warm water may also relax tight muscles and tendons.

WHAT IS THE RECOMMENDED DOSAGE?

The standard recommended daily dose of magnesium is 400 mg a day. My experience is that higher doses are sometimes necessary for a consistent pharmacologic effect. This is why it is important to work with a doctor who is knowledgeable about natural substances like magnesium and their effective doses and use.

Different people experience varying degrees of side effects with magnesium. It can cause considerable difficulty with intestinal discomfort or diarrhea. Many types of laxatives work because they contain magnesium. I tried many types of magnesium, even at low doses, and still developed problems. Ultimately I found one that worked for me: Magnesium Plus Protein. It contains simple magnesium oxide, which is considered a rather crude form of the substance, but it was wrapped in a protein base that facilitated its absorption. It worked for me, and because my disease was so severe, I was happy to have found it. It wasn't the type of magnesium that mattered, but the ability to absorb it and obtain its consistent benefit.

Moreover, we must also wonder why people taking FQs became magnesium deficient while taking the antibiotics. Is it then essential for these people to take magnesium to restore balance to their systems, including enough magnesium to begin healing again? This might explain why so many people with FTS heal so slowly. This must be studied and determined as soon as we can. It is one of the most important questions of this book.

Although I do not recommend the high dosage of magnesium I took for so many years, it is often necessary to take increased dosages such as 600, 800, or perhaps 1,000 mg a day for months. Alternative practitioners often prescribe these types of doses for hypertension or migraines, and it would not be surprising if they are necessary for many months to promote healing of FTS. And a major corollary of this thinking is to also urge the FDA to discover a method of measuring, accurately, blood levels of magnesium in humans. This would greatly help us measure the level of this vital substance in people.

When magnesium is given intravenously, such as for acute migraines, it may take 1,000 or 2,000 mg of magnesium IV to break the migraine attack. The body usually excretes the extra magnesium quickly in the urine. That is why it is also important to drink plenty of water when taking magnesium. Because magnesium is usually excreted quickly via the kidneys, it is better to take the supplement in divided doses during the day. This approach allows your body to maintain a magnesium level for much of the day, thereby providing magnesium for tissue repair and restoration.

Work closely with your healthcare advisor to determine your proper daily dose of magnesium, especially if you have kidney failure. Be sure your advisor checks your magnesium level every month or so. I checked my magnesium levels many times and they were always normal. I did very well on the supplement for fifteen years. The daily doses were higher than I liked, but necessary to control the severe pain. Nevertheless, I ultimately developed side effects, including a tremor, instability in my walking, and somewhat slurred speech. I had to discontinue the magnesium in favor of other therapies, and the side effects slowly went away.

It had taken a very large intake of magnesium on a daily basis for many years to develop an overuse disorder. I tested my magnesium levels dozens of times over the years, and even when my toxicity became apparent, my blood tests were normal. Magnesium is an intracellular substance, and it tends to build up within the central nervous system. Even though the blood levels may look fine, they may still be high. The cessation of my magnesium led to the disappearance of my neurological symptoms, thus proving that the magnesium was the culprit. My blood tests remained normal even then, when I hadn't taken any magnesium supplements or magnesium-rich foods for a year.

CONCLUSION

If you have FTS, taking magnesium is imperative for healing, so work with a knowledgeable healthcare professional who knows about this vital mineral. Better yet, use it when you first take a FQ. It is helpful to think that the use of magnesium might allow us to prevent FTS as soon as it shows signs of occurring. And to hope that using magnesium as described will also allow us to use FQs when these drugs are truly needed as effective antibiotics without injuring so many so badly.

7

The Benefits of N-Acetylcysteine, Zinc, and Vitamin E

This chapter discusses three different substances which have been proven in recent studies to help treat the effects of fluoroquinolone toxicity syndrome: N-acetylcysteine, zinc, and vitamin E. Like magnesium, all three are available at the drug store for purchase without a doctor's prescription. Evidence on the benefits of N-acetylcysteine, zinc, and vitamin E for fluoroquinolone toxicity is still preliminary, but promising nonetheless. Consult your healthcare advisor about the possibility of using these medications for treating fluoroquinolone toxicity.

CAN N-ACETYLCYSTEINE HELP PREVENT FTS?

Using magnesium to block the oxidative damage, mitochondrial dysfunction, and DNA injury caused by FQs has promise, but it is not simple to do. Using magnesium for infusion therapy to block FTS onset seems to have promise for people with symptoms of FTS, as in Sean's case in Chapter 6. But there are difficulties in applying this approach, and most doctors are not knowledgeable about magnesium and have little interest in using it orally or intravenously. Is there another safe substance that might be used?

I never thought I would be able to answer this questions with a yes, but in July 2013 an important study by Kalghati et al. was published in the medical journal *Science Translational Medicine*. The article described the degree of oxidative damage to DNA, proteins, and cellular membrane lipids that can occur when these cellular factors are exposed to bactericidal antibiotics, including FQs. Most important, the deleterious effects of the bactericidal antibiotics, including Cipro, "were alleviated in

73

[human] cell culture and in mice by the administration of the antioxidant N-acetylcysteine."

Does this mean that we might have an additional option to protect people from tissue injury when they are prescribed FQs for a serious infection? And can this option be used at the very same time people take their FQs, unlike magnesium, which must be used hours away from FQ therapy?

What is N-Acetylcysteine?

N-acetylcysteine (NAC) is a natural substance produced by the human body in small quantities. It is developed from the chemical bonding of the part of a molecule known as an *acetyl group* to the amino acid *cysteine.* Acetyl groups plays many roles in human chemical processes, including the Krebs cycle, which generates energy for the respiration that all cells perform. One well known acetyl is acetyl salicylic acid, or ASA—otherwise known as aspirin.

Hence, we have N-Acetyl-Cysteine. Cysteine is a semi-essential amino acid, meaning is natural to the human body. In human cells, NAC is known for restoring our levels of glutathione, the substance key to human cells in balancing the cellular system against the destructive effect of reactive oxygen species (ROS), or excessive oxidation. One of the primary mechanisms by which FQs injure human tissues and impair healing is from intense levels of oxidants. For many years, infusions of glutathione were recommended as a method of treating FTS by blocking ROS impact on cells. In this way, glutathione was said to promote the healing of tissues injured by FTS. But in actuality, the benefits of glutathione infusions for FTS were mixed at best.

In 2004, Rob developed FTS while taking eight pills of Avelox (moxifloxacin).

"I became so horribly damaged that I did not think I would ever recover," he told me. After showing little improvement for two years, Rob slowly recovered by about 90 percent, according to him and his wife. Rob was able to return to work. I also spoke to Rob's doctor, who agreed with Rob's assessment. This degree of improvement after two years of disability was impressive. It was never entirely clear whether Rob's improvement was due to the glutathione infusions or simply due to the body's healing itself over a long period of time. Still, Rob had made little progress in the years before the glutathione treatment. After my report, several others tried glutathione infusions, but their results were less impressive. However, their courses of glutathione were much shorter than Rob's.

NAC is a legitimate medical therapy. For decades, it has been used by people with heavy colds to break up the congestion in their chests. Others with conditions such as cystic fibrosis use inhalers or steamers with NAC to break up the thick mucus in their lungs. NAC is also used in emergency rooms and hospitals for people who have made suicide attempts with acetaminophen (Tylenol), a powerful liver toxin. Similar medical situations sometimes occur with people who take too much acetaminophen not knowing the substance has been contaminated in many combination pain medications. Other times, people have taken excessive doses of acetaminophen because they assume it is perfectly safe, being an over-the-counter drug. Many people were not aware of its lethal capability. For decades, acetaminophen has been the leading cause of death from toxic liver failure in America. Some years ago, the recommended doses were reduced, a long overdue change.

NAC has properties that can block other inflammatory processes in cells that can cause pain and cellular damage. NAC is said to block DNA damage and possibly prevent the development of some cancers. Recent studies suggest that NAC can protect against insulin resistance seen in obesity. It can, to some degree, reduce the inflammatory symptoms seen with seasonal flu, and reduce the inflammation with the gastritis that occurs with gastric helicobacter pylori infections, which are a common cause of stomach ulcers.

The medicinal properties of NAC are well-known by integrative and alternative practitioners. According to the 2013 study discussed above, NAC's beneficial properties may extend to reducing the severe reactions with FQs that have injured or permanently impaired tens of thousands of people.

Evidence for NAC

In the 2013 study mentioned above, one of the authors' main questions was: Can a FQ, such as Cipro, be used together with NAC without interfering with the effectiveness of the antibiotic? This would be a major breakthrough in trying to curb the Cipro catastrophe. Their answer:

> We showed that reactive oxidative species and oxidative damage induced by bacterial antibiotics could be abrogated while having little

effect on the killing efficacy of these antibiotics on bacteria. The concentration of NAC used to reduce antibiotic-induced oxidative damage
in mammalian cells did not decrease the bacterial killing efficacy.

This is a major finding! In other words, the antibiotic remained effective, while NAC's impact on the host cells (i.e., the human cells) was protective. Overall, these findings suggest that using NAC at the same time
as a FQ would not compromise the antibiotic's activity. NAC is far superi-
or to magnesium, which cannot be used at the very same time as a FQ. In
other words, NAC might go a long way to minimizing the damage caused
to human structures by FQs. NAC could possibly reduce the impact of the
ROS from FQs, as well as reduce FQ injuries caused to the mitochondria
and DNA, as seen in human cell culture.

Based on this study, it seems NAC treatment might be undertaken
quickly, at the first sign of FQs. The doctor might start NAC with a patient
at the very same time the FQ is started. This might allow treatment of the
patient's infection while protecting the patient from a reaction to the FQ.
The NAC could be continued after the FQ has been stopped. Remember, there have been many reports of FQ reactions days, weeks, or even
months after discontinuing FQs. Best known have been late occurrences of sudden Achilles tendon ruptures six months after a FQ has been
discontinued.

The researchers also induced a urinary tract infection in mice and
treated them with Cipro alone or with Cipro in combination with NAC.
This was an important aspect of their investigation, because it was tested
whether the NAC would alter the Cipro's effectiveness in treating the
infection. It did not. The presence of the NAC in the mice's bodies did not
interfere with the Cipro's effectiveness against the urinary tract infection.
This was a key finding.

In previous studies, some antioxidants impacted bactericidal antibiotics and diminished their effectiveness. One of these was glutathione,
which had been shown to reduce the efficacy of bactericidal antibiotics.
Magnesium could also be a problem. But it appears that NAC can be used
during FQ antibiotic therapy without interfering with the Cipro's antibacterial effect, while NAC proceeds with reducing oxidative damage, ROS
overproduction, and mitochondrial dysfunction.

The standard recommended dosage of NAC is 600 mg taken as an
antioxidant three times daily. In everyday use, people often take one, two,
or three NAC daily. The specific human dosage suggested from this study

was not defined. For severe symptoms of emerging FTS, intravenous NAC may be considered at the higher doses used for acute Tylenol overdose. Discuss this with your doctor or with a pain specialist. The authors also suggested that the increased incidence of FTS in people over sixty, as the FDA states, "may be the result of falling levels of glutathione that occurs with advancing age." In other words, older people with FTS may need higher doses of NAC.

The important findings of this study need to be confirmed as soon as possible. In the previous three chapters, I discussed the large body of information on magnesium and FQs. I believe that magnesium is still important in the prevention and treatment of FTS. Still, problems with absorption and possible interactions create some complications that need to be studied and solved. So while the use of magnesium and FQs is still being determined, NAC seems to have few of magnesium's complications, so its use might be considered right away. At the same time, studies should be undertaken immediately by FQ manufacturers and at medical institutions to determine how we might best use NAC in people requiring FQ therapy. It would be wonderful to find a substance that can protect human DNA and mitochondria when FQs are used today and in the future.

One of my big questions is whether we should start studying the use and safety of people with FTS and in those given FQs. A mainstream doctor may not know much about NAC but hopefully will have an open mind. Knowing NAC's wide use for Tylenol overdoses, your doctor may be swayed by NAC's possible benefits. Your alternative healthcare practitioner might welcome this new information and be willing to work with you. We have all been waiting and hoping for a breakthrough. NAC is well-known, safe, and effective, and with a long history of use for many serious conditions. Our healthcare system must get going on these types of studies.

Because NAC is available at health food stores and at vitamin websites, you don't really need anyone's permission to take it to help prevent FTS. The big question is whether we have enough data to know if it might work. We don't. We need studies on NAC, magnesium, and the many other medications and supplements with the potential to treat or prevent FTS. If something like NAC might work, and it has had decades of safety testing in humans, it seems the risk ratio is low and the safety benefit might be very high in reducing the terrible scourge of FTS. We also know from a few small studies that vitamin E and zinc might be useful. This is the FDA's chance to take the lead and light our way.

VITAMIN E

In Chapter 7, I discussed the 2007 study that showed us that rats fed a diet with vitamin E supplementation before being given Cipro had a 41 percent reduction in cartilage injuries in comparison to a second group of rats given Cipro without supplements in their diet beforehand. A third group of rats fed a diet with magnesium supplementation before given Cipro had a 65 percent reduction in cartilage injuries when compared to the second group of rats given Cipro without any additional supplementation. In other words, the supplement led to a substantial reduction in cartilage injuries in the rats. These reductions were highly significant.

Even more significant was the 82 percent reduction in cartilage injuries in the fourth group of rats given feed with both vitamin E and magnesium supplementation for seven days before given Cipro. Such a treatment course is not practical for people needing an antibiotic right away, which is often the case for antibiotic therapy. And although we already know that magnesium can bind to FQs, we don't know whether vitamin E would be a problem. Such an incompatibility would be unlikely, yet none of the materials about FQs say anything about an incompatibility with magnesium, which we know exists. So this needs to be studied regarding vitamin E. Can it be taken safely at the same time as a FQ, or must the supplement be taken hours apart from the FQ?

A 2006 study showed that in cell culture, vitamin E provided partial protection from FQ damage to DNA. In fact, when the authors of this study published it in *Neurotoxicology*, they wrote:

> The mechanism of these adverse effects [gastrointestinal, central nervous system, and dermatological] has not yet been elucidated. The aim of this study was to investigate the possible DNA damage-inducing effect of a fluoroquinolone antibiotic, ciprofloxacin, on primary culture of rat astrocytes. ... Our results showed a concentration-dependent induction of DNA damage ... Pretreatment of cells with vitamin E for four hours provided partial protection from this effect.

Vitamin E's benefit is likely from the supplement's powerful antioxidant effect. Use the d-alpha form of vitamin E tocepherols instead of the less potent, synthetic dl-alpha form. The usual recommended dosage of vitamin E is 200 IU once or twice a day. Excessive vitamin E can increase a bleeding tendency, so people taking Coumadin (warfarin), Plavix (clopidogrel), Pradaxa (dabigatran etexilate), or any of the other anticoagulation drugs, omega-3 oils, ginkgo biloba, or another blood thinning supplement should discuss these with their healthcare advisors.

Another idea that you should consider trying is a mix of vitamin E and NAC together. The combination might boost each supplement's protective benefits against FQ toxicity or FTS. We already know that NAC has been shown to have no complications when used at the same time as a FQ. Vitamin E might provide additional protection to human cells when a FQ is being used. Ideas like these must be studied as soon and as thoroughly as possible.

ZINC

Zinc is a trace mineral in the human body essential for the proper functioning of enzymes and their involvement in the cell processes. Zinc participates in the regulation of gene expression, protein activity, and immunity. Zinc is included as a component of total parenteral nutrition in patients with severe malnutrition, and for improving outcomes with burn patients.

A study, published in 2012, describes injuries due to oxidative stress from a FQ and the impact on cartilage and bone, as well as on DNA in rats. The authors found that "Administration of magnesium, zinc chloride, and vitamin E were found to prevent or reverse ciprofloxacin-induced chrondrotoxicity and tendinopathy in animals. … Further evaluation of these antioxidants' effect in ciprofloxacin-induced chrondrotoxicity and tendinopathy in humans could be of clinical importance as observed in many animal studies." Please note the researchers' use of the words "were found to prevent or *reverse*." This is not a word commonly used in discussing FTS. Let's make a note.

Another study of zinc was performed by Channa, Ashfag, Bangash, Abbasi, and Qureshi in 2008. The purpose was to assess the preventative role of zinc chloride on the cartilage toxicity produced by ciprofloxacin in a young Wistar albino rat litter. This was a prospective study, a very high quality form of study. It found that "simultaneous zinc chloride administration minimized the epiphyseal cartilage damage induced by ciprofloxacin."

The United States and United Kingdom health agencies recommend 10 mg a day of zinc for men and 7 mg a day for women. Many mineral formulas contain 10 or 15 mg of zinc a day. The body does not store zinc, so a daily dosage is advisable.

CONCLUSION

The studies conducted on the value of NAC, vitamin E, and zinc for treating fluoroquinolone toxicity are a start, but we must keep looking for ideas and answers. Now is the time for our medical and pharmaceutical and alternative systems to move strongly forward and to take decisive steps toward solving FTS for the tens of thousands who have been impacted.

8

Tried and True Remedies

This chapter presents oral therapies that have been reported to provide varying degrees of benefit for FTS. Unlike the four substances discussed in the previous chapters, the therapies in this chapter have not been studied systematically for FTS. In my opinion, nothing discussed in this chapter is earth-shattering or will stop FTS. Most of the reports in this chapter are patient-based and are meant to provide pain relief or medical assistance. They have been found helpful by one or a few people. If you are interested in some of them, I suggest discussing them with your healthcare advisor.

Responses of individuals can vary. If you are concerned about side effects, start with low doses, such as one-half or one-quarter the standard amount or less. In my practice, I saw many people with histories of medication sensitivities. Unless the situation was an emergency, I often started these people at low doses. If the low dose was inadequate, I increased the amount gradually until an effective dosage was reached. This approach is known as *dosage titration*, that is, gradually adjusting the dosage to fit the individual's tolerance and need. It can work quite well, but you can apply this approach only to medications for human systems, not for drugs, cancers, or infections.

DISCUSS WITH YOUR DOCTOR

Doctors need to position themselves as intermediaries for their medically injured patients. They should be open and interested in the feedback from patients and curious about legitimate side effects that their patients identify. Doctors must be ready to challenge drug company representatives who are often uninformed about a new drug's risks. Patients and doctors are often unaware of how little is known about powerful new drugs like FQs when they are first approved. If a patient seems credible, why not consider what he or she is saying? It's quite common for side effects to be missed during prerelease research and only recognized when given to the general population long after the drug was approved. Many advances in the history of medicine were initiated only after thoughtful patients experienced an unexpected reaction to a new drug. Indeed, formal definitions of "evidence-based medicine," the modern term for reliable medical knowledge, include anecdotal reports from patients as legitimate sources of medical information.

At my first job as a doctor at a university medical clinic, I heard many women complain about their menstrual migraines, abdominal pains, or low energy. The medical authorities dismissed these complaints outright and recommended that these "hysterical" women be given strange drug combinations that contained barbiturates, amphetamines, aspirin, and diuretics, top sellers at the time. Many of these women were bright, emotionally steady, consistent in their stories, and didn't want to take the drugs. All of this was apparent to me after just thirty seconds of listening to them. I became convinced their complaints were legitimate. Yet, for decades doctors were trained to view these women as hysterical, needy, or drug-seeking. That's when I first learned how easily doctors resort to the blame-the-patient tactics when patients raise complains that the medical profession doesn't want to hear or understand. We have been doing the very same thing today, denying complaints about FTS.

That's not to say that all FTS complaints are reliable. As with any complaints of side effects, some are accurate and some probably are not. The important part is that a patient's input may sometimes provide a starting point for identifying problems missed or ignored in early drug company testing. And while it is true that people suffering FTS may be of different ages or genders, learning which therapies helped one person with FTS may be instructive for others. Even if ten anecdotal reports prove unhelpful, the eleventh may provide a clue useful to others with FTS. Formal definitions of evidence-based medicine agree about the usefulness of information from various sources.

Drug companies have spent billions to convince doctors that clinical trials are the only worthwhile form of medical proof. They call these

R.L.'s Protocol

Information from patients can sometimes prove useful for others having similar trouble, particularly because the medical-pharmaceutical complex has not studied these problems in FTS. Although FTS has been caused by the pharmaceutical industry, the companies have shown little interest in studying the problem and possible solutions. When I first spoke to R.L. several years ago, his FTS consisted primarily of tendon and muscle pain, as well as some neurological systems and a nasty sleep disorder. He decided to conduct his own study, and contacted me a year later to tell me that he had gained significant improvement. He credits the following:

1. **Magnesium citrate** 325 mg twice daily, and **magnesium aspartate** 250 mg once per day.

2. **Turmeric, an anti-inflammatory.** R.L. wrote, "I stopped limping after taking turmeric for a month or so."

3. **Taurine,** 300 mg a day. "I understand this helps magnesium absorption." Opinions vary on this.

4. **Methylcobalamin, a form of B-12** said to be better absorbed than standard hydroxycobalamin. R.L.'s dosage: sublingual B-12 5,000 mcg a day, far beyond the minimum required dosage of 2.5 to 5 micrograms per day.

5. **Melatonin,** 25 mg in the evening, sometimes taken with a B-vitamin complex.

6. **Vitamin D3,** 5,000 IU a day.

NOTE: R.L. took a total magnesium dose of 900 mg a day, exceeding the recommended dietary allowance (RDA). My experience is that individuals do well on different magnesium regiments. Higher doses of magnesium often are required for pharmacologic effect. Be sure to discuss the importance of magnesium for FTS, as well as the type and dosage, with your health advisor. Obtain regular blood levels, perhaps bimonthly. Drink sufficient liquids each day and discuss your other supplements with your healthcare advisor.

studies the "gold standard." Such marketing is designed to convince doctors that only drugs are worthy of consideration. A distinct corollary of this viewpoint are the doctors' refusals to believe that drugs can cause serious side effects, as we have seen with FQs. No wonder so many doctors remain skeptical about the many serious warnings the FDA has issued for FQs.

If you firmly believe that you have been injured by a FQ, you should still allow your doctor to perform a thorough medical evaluation with a spectrum of blood tests, MRIs, EMGs (for detecting some, but not all, nerve injuries). It is important for both you and your doctor to have some confidence that reasonable diagnostic possibilities have been considered. Many doctors unfamiliar with FTS might think you have an autoimmune or neurological or endocrine disorder. It is appropriate to have these possibilities eliminated. For example, FQs can trigger acute anxiety and panic disorder, but so can an overactive thyroid gland or an adrenal dysfunction. Better to have important medical conditions ruled out so that you are guided in the right direction.

TREATMENTS FOR PAIN WITH ORAL THERAPIES

Severe, long-term pain from FTS often keeps people from working, exercising, and from everyday use of their bodies. Chronic pain can drain people emotionally and lead to depression and despair. It should be treated whenever possible.

Turmeric (Curcumin)

Turmeric is probably the best known nondrug supplement with substantial anti-inflammatory effect. The main ingredient in turmeric is curcumin, along with two other curcuminoids: dimethoxycurcumin and bisdemethoxycurcumin. Absorption of turmeric after oral intake is poor. Dosing twice or three times a day may be necessary to obtain a consistent anti-inflammatory effect.

Studies in animals and humans have suggested that curcumin may be helpful for reducing inflammation in rheumatoid arthritis, ulcerative colitis, Crohn's disease, pancreatitis, osteoarthritis, anteriti uveitis of the eye, and other inflammatory disorders. In addition, research has been undertaken on curcumin for its potential anticancer effect. The most common adverse effect reported with curcumin is gastrointestinal irritation. Curcumin supplements often vary in their concentration and daily dosage. Ask your natural healthcare provider.

Boswellia

Gleaned from Boswellia species in Africa and India, this natural anti-inflammatory herb has been used for millennia in Ayurvedic medicine. Boswellia is often used for arthritis, inflammatory bowel diseases, and asthma. The scientific evidence for boswellia's therapeutic effect is good. As with turmeric, products with boswellia can vary in their concentrations and dosages, and a common adverse effect is stomach discomfort.

Anti-Inflammatory Medications (NSAIDs)

Many individuals are uncomfortable with using anti-inflammatory drugs (NSAIDs) because of the FDA's stern warning against mixing them with FQs: "Taking an NSAID while you take Cipro or other fluoroquinolones may increase your risk of central nervous system effects and seizures." Some people interpret this warning to mean that taking NSAIDs at any time after suffering from toxic effects is risky. However, others interpret this warning to mean that the two types of drugs should not be taken at the same time. In other words, there appears to be no extra risk if an NSAID is taken in moderation long after FQs have been discontinued.

Some patients have done well with NSAIDs, and others have not. Of course, NSAIDs can cause side effects such as stomach pain. One of my patients did well with Aleve (naproxen) when she used it intermittently for her musculoskeletal pains. It helped her gradually become active and eventually return to work. She did not take the naproxen constantly, but only when needed. Still, to be safe and to not have to worry, check with your doctor or pharmacist.

We know that NSAIDs can increase the risk of heart attacks. My understanding is that naproxen (Aleve, Naprosyn) is one of the safest NSAIDs, and ibuprofen (Motrin) is close behind in safety. Again, some people do well on different NSAIDs. To improve safety, start with an OTC dosage. Dosage is a key factor in determining the risk of medications. Just like with alcohol, the lower the dose, the lower the risk. You want to use a dose large enough to obtain a drug's benefit, but no larger than needed. Other times you may need a prescription dose to obtain a sufficient benefit. Remember: the best dose of any medication is the least amount that you require for it to work. Excessive doses bring more risk.

Cortisone (Steroids)

The FDA strongly warns doctors to avoid prescribing corticosteroids (e.g., predisone, prednisolone, and many others) for patients who are taking FQ medications. Why? Because when used together, both can increase the risk of tendon ruptures. Even long after a FQ is discontinued, steroids alone can increase the risk of developing a ruptured tendon. Instances of this happening have been reported in the medical literature many times.

Still, steroid therapy has been used with FTS when doctors believe the condition is autoimmune in nature or when the doctor is trying to reduce the patient's level of inflammation or pain. This approach is not advised with a FQ. The risk persists with FQs and steroids even months after the FQ is discontinued.

In my 2001 survey of people developing neuropathies with FQs, ten people stated that they had received steroids for their FQ-related symptoms, and five reported improvement. Two reported worsening. A few years later, a man contacted my office to say that low-dose steroid therapy had produced marked improvement in his tendon pain. If you are considering this approach, be sure to discuss with your doctor the potential benefits and risks, including tendon rupture, of using steroids for FTS.

Muscle Relaxants

Sarah developed FTS soon after being prescribed Levaquin for a urinary tract infection. The infection had a few symptoms and may not have warranted treatment in the first place. This happens a lot in everyday medical care. Powerful drugs like Cipro or other FQs are used for garden variety conditions that can be treated more mildly and safely. In fact, I have come to believe that FQs should almost never be used as the first line treatment for a bladder or sinus infection. There are many other effective antibiotics with far fewer risks that can be used quite effectively. As the medical journals are starting to show, many doctors are beginning to believe the same thing.

Sarah's symptoms were FQ side effects, mainly musculoskeletal in nature, and although her X-rays and MRIs were normal, she had considerable pain, arriving at my office using crutches to carry her weight. Fearful of medications but not helped by the supplements she was taking, we started with a tiny amount of anti-inflammatory medication: 81 mg baby aspirin tablet two or three times a day. This provided an adequate amount of anti-inflammatory effect. Also useful was 5 mg of Valium at bedtime that relaxed her muscles and facilitated her sleep through the night. This low-dose regimen kept her comfortable for several months while her aching body showed gradual improvement. Although some people experience prolonged FTS, many others exhibit improvement within a few weeks or months. Three months later, Sarah returned without her crutches.

Muscle relaxants can be helpful for patients with muscle pain or tight tendons. There are many types of prescription muscle relaxants, such as Zanaflex (tizanidine), Flexeril (cyprobenzaprine), Robaxin (methocarbamol), and Soma (carisoprodol). Other people have tried benzodiazepines like Valium (diazepam) and Klonopin (clonazepam), which can facilitate muscle relaxation and sleep. Although these medications can be sedating to some people when used during the day, others do not experience this. Ask your healthcare advisor about how to use these medications in order to obtain benefit without dependency.

There are a few natural supplements that can be helpful for pain or tight muscles. The best known are GABA and theanine, substances you can find at health food stores. They can help reduce anxiety, promote muscle relaxation, and improve sleep. They come in a range of doses. Similar supplements, such as kava or melatonin, can improve relaxation. Trytophan can be used for promoting sleep, as can its metabolite, 5-hydroxy-trytophan (5-HTP). In some people, tryptophan and 5-HTP can have antidepressant effects or can cause unusual dreams.

Tramadol (Ultram)

This pain medication has dual action as a weak opioid analgesic (similar in strength to codeine) and also as a mild serotonin and norepinephrine reuptake inhibitor. One patient with years of pain from FTS, Barbara, was helped substantially with low doses of tramadol. We watched her dosage carefully, and I had her skip the tramadol when she didn't need it, thereby avoiding overuse or tolerance. Other patients use medications such as NSAIDs or opiates similarly, very carefully and only when needed. For sure, people injured by FTS are leery of drugs, reluctant to use them, and when they do, it is usually done carefully.

Antidepressants

Cymbalta (duloxetine) is used to treat many conditions: depression, neuropathic pain (e.g., diabetic neuropathies), and also fibromyalgia, chronic musculoskeletal pain, and the osteoarthritis of aging. Cymbalta and Effexor work similarly by increasing the neurotransmitters serotonin and norepinephrine. These drugs are sometimes well-tolerated by patients, but other patients sometimes find them to be harsh. When I first met Scott, age forty-eight, he had already been severely disabled by FTS for more than a year. Scott had been physically active for years in a lacrosse league previous to using FQs. He also had a physically taxing job. When disabled by FTS, Scott could hardly walk and remained in bed for most of the day. He had to quit his job and sport. He suffered continual pain and became very depressed.

After much discussion, Scott and I agreed to try Cymbalta, starting

How Low Can a Medication Go?

From the first pharmacology class in medical school, I was enchanted. The type of thinking that pharmacology required fit my brain perfectly. Here is one of the cases that grabbed me. I found it in a top reference book, the *United States Pharmacopoeia*, one of the great resources going back decades. I used to browse it for fun.

A woman had Mediterranean fever, a genetic disorder affecting protein production in the body and causing severe inflammation in many organs. It was a difficult condition to treat in the late 2000s. Sometimes it was lethal. By far, the best medication for Mediterranean fever was **colchicine,** an old-time drug notorious for causing side effects. Colchicine could cause severe stomach pain, cramping, and diarrhea in as many as 80 percent of patients. Part of the problem was that colchicine was made from a crude herb and came in only one size. All patients received the same dosage. Could it be that the dosage was simply too strong for some patients?

Colchicine made this particular woman very sick, but she had a creative physician who understood the importance of individualizing each patient's with a low dosage, one-quarter of a capsule per day. For some people, Cymbalta can be a powerful drug and it can take them a while to adapt. As we gradually increased Scott's dosage to the standard amount of 20 mg per morning, Scott's pain dropped and his mood improved. Orthopedic evaluations showed no major injuries to his tendons or joints. Scott's movement improved. His physical therapy, which focused on lower abdominal tendon mobilization, continued to gain ground. I encouraged Scott to use codeine or Aleve if needed intermittently for pain. These allowed him to gradually increase his activity, which was important for him physically and psychologically. Improving slowly, not pushing himself beyond his capabilities, Scott became improved enough to return to work after a year. When I last saw him, Scott still had pain from FTS and was unable to return to lacrosse, but he was walking better, working full-time, and he was hopeful that his physical activities would continue to improve.

Effexor (venlafaxine) is similar to Cymbalta, but I have often preferred Effexor for some of my patients because it was easier for me to adjust

dosage. The doctor understood that if he started her at a low enough dosage, in time she might adjust to her medication. By doing so, she might obtain some medication benefit without serious side effects. The doctor started this woman with the lowest medication dosage I have ever heard: .001 mg, which was 1/600th of the standard starting colchicine dose. He then increased the dose very gradually. Three months later, the woman reached the full, necessary dosage her condition required.

If you start patients low enough and go forward slowly enough, almost any person can be treated with any medication (assuming they are not allergic to it). I've had some patients start at one-quarter and even one-tenth the standard starting dosages of drugs. With time, the medication dosage can usually be raised gradually. Sometimes a gradual dose escalation is not necessary, because very low doses are sufficient for some people. I have been amazed at times, but then I realize that if drug responses can vary up to 4,000 percent from one person to the next, as the American Medical Association has long stated, then just about anything is possible.

dose to fit some of my patients' medication sensitivities. Throughout my medical career dating back to the 1970s, I have met many people who were unusually sensitive to the potency or side effects of medications like antidepressants. My approach has always been to follow the FDA advice and "start low, go slow." This applied most often to women and seniors. Unless a medication reaction is an emergency, starting low is usually the safer, milder route.

For example, the standard starting dose of Effexor is most often 75 or 150 mg in a long-acting capsule. Sometimes this approach works very well. But for some patients, especially those with histories of sensitivity to medications, I started at a 50 mg or 37.5 mg tablet of Effexor. There is even a 25 mg size of Effexor, and for those with long histories of medication reactions, I will sometimes start a patient with one-half of this dosage (12.5 mg). When patients understand that the goal is not speed, but safety, they feel greatly reassured that they will not be rushed into higher and higher, stronger and stronger doses that will cause undesirable side effects.

Drug companies teach doctors that patients must meet specific dosages in order to obtain benefit. But this has not proven true in many of my patients. When Prozac was released in 1988, the lowest dose produced was 20 mg daily. The drug worked extremely well for some people, but others developed severe side effects. I went to the UCSD biomedical library and scanned the stacks (no computers yet!) Early research revealed that at a lower dose of 5 mg of Prozac, 54 percent of seriously depressed people improved considerably. Equally important, side effects were much less frequent and fewer people quit treatment. The lesson was and remains that the key in using medications with patients is matching the right drug at the right dosage to the right patient. Pharmacists have been adhering to this clinical dictum for a century. After their experience with FTS, people are often frightened by the idea of side effects from medications, and they feel much more comfortable starting with a low dose of a drug.

TREATMENT POSSIBILITIES FOR PERIPHERAL NEUROPATHIES

The peripheral nervous system is one of the most frequent systems affected by FTS. As discussed in Chapter 3, the FDA cites many peripheral neuropathy symptoms in FTS such as burning, tingling, or heat sensations;

numbness; and weakness or pain involving the arms, hands, legs, or feet. These symptoms range from subtle and mild to severe or intense.

The medical evaluation and tests of the peripheral neuropathies from FTS may not be revealing because peripheral nerves are usually tiny and difficult to evaluate. When doctors order nerve studies such as the electromyography (EMG), these tests typically examine the larger nerves deeper in the trunk and limbs. However, such smaller studies do not always find pathology in the small nerve fibers. Sometimes, this may be misleading because FTS to smaller fiber neuropathies can be undetectable on standard nerve tests. The injuries may be there, but our usual methods of diagnosing small fiber neuropathies with EMG may have difficult indentifying them. To tell people with significant peripheral nerve injuries from FTS that there's nothing wrong with them may be misleading. One person's doctor understood this and ordered a punch biopsy of the skin in the area of his symptoms. This approach allowed the abnormal nerve fibers to be seen microscopically. Ask your doctor if this approach might be useful in identifying your signs of nervous system FTS.

Some medications can be helpful for peripheral neuropathies. These include Cymbalta and Effexor, which I have discussed previously. As I mentioned, they have been approved for this use by the FDA.

Gabapentin

Gabapentin, or by its brand name, Neurontin, is a nerve pain medication and anticonvulsant. When first started, gabapentin can cause drowsiness, lightheadedness, or dizziness. Most doctors start with 300 mg orally three times a day, but if you are sensitive to medications, you might start with 100 mg three times a day. Often the dosage is increased gradually to as much as 600 mg three times daily or higher. In some people, gabapentin can wear off before the next dosage. For this event, long-acting form of gabapentin has recently been released. It usually is begun at the low dosage of 300, and can be gradually increased to as high as 1,800 mg. This long-acting form, usually taken with dinner, is called Gralise.

Pregabalin

Another commonly prescribed anticonvulsant and nerve pain medication is Lyrica, which can be quite effective, but other times it may cause side effects that necessitate discontinuance. Other drugs typically used for seizures or other neurological disorders have been used successfully for neuropathies. For example, the Mayo Clinic lists other anti-seizure medications such as Topamax (topiramate), Tegretol (carbamezapine), and Dilantin (phenytoin). Tricylic antidepressants, such as Elavil (amitriptyline), Sinequan (doxepin), and Parmelor (nortriptyline) can be quite effective for peripheral neuropathies, but have many side effects. You can find more information at the Mayo Clinic website, mayoclinic.org.

Natural Supplements for Neuropathies

Treatment of peripheral neuropathies can vary from person to person. Some people have good experiences with medications, but others experience minimal relief or have many side effects. In general, I have done better overall with natural remedies for neuropathies. I first learned about these alternative methods when I developed reflex sympathetic dystrophy. In 1998 I learned that *alpha lipoic acid* (ALA), a natural element, could be quite helpful at times. Some experts who dispense natural therapies recommend intravenous infusions of ALA once or twice a week. This can be a powerful therapy. My experience has been different. Because my disorder has been a chronic, day-by-day condition, I found that over time, using ALA (also known as L-ALA) multiple times each day was more effective and consistent, and helped in my getting well around 2007.

I also found that regular ALA has always worked better for me than R-ALA, a newer form that is recommended by some nutriceutical suppliers. Using standard ALA every few hours all day long has been one of my most effective therapies. It has taken me a while to figure this approach out. Yes, it can become tedious having to use this substance so frequently, but pain relief is a powerful source of reward. The usual recommended dosage of ALA is 400 mg four times a day, but a dose of 200 mg every two hours works better for me. Go figure. Check with your integrative healthcare provider.

The other supplement that has helped my severe neuropathies has been magnesium. I have discussed my use of oral magnesium and its dosage previously. Some people have found mild baths with *magnesium sulfate* crystals—otherwise known as Epsom salt—to be quite helpful. This is available at many pharmacies without prescription. For me, oral supplementation has always worked better. We are all different, and so are our medical conditions, including those with different types of FTS.

Another effective supplement for neuropathies is an advanced derivative of thiamine known as *benfontamine.* Whereas a high dose of thiamine is 100 mg, benfontamine has been used effectively and safely at 600 or even 1,200 mg per day. It is often used 100 or 200 mg at a time, multiple times a day. *Acetyl-L-carnitine* is yet another good supplement that has been effective for neuropathies by alternative practitioners. I have had two patients whose neuropathies displayed marked improvement with this substance. Dosage is usually 150 or 500 mg three or four times a day. The most common adverse effect of acetyl-L-carintine for these patients was gastritis, which can be reduced by taking it with food, ginger, or over-the-counter or prescription ranitidine (Zantac) or omeprazole (Prilosec).

TREATMENT FOR SLEEP DISORDERS

Disturbed sleep is a common feature of FTS and should be treated, if possible. I am not a sleep specialist, but I know that persistent sleep is essential. Meditation, guided muscle relaxation, or guided imagery can often be helpful for this problem. If these don't work, sleep is important enough to resort to natural or medicinal remedies, when necessary. *Melatonin* is the natural compound the brain produces and secretes to tell the body to go to sleep. Available as a supplement in most drug stores, melatonin is a popular, natural sleep aid that helps many people achieve restful sleep. Health store employees often know about melatonin and a variety of other natural supplements, herbs, or natural combinations for sleep. Don't hesitate to ask questions.

Standard pharmacies are now carrying some sleep combinations with natural supplements and herbs. This is a good trend. One popular combination remedy contains valerian root extract, theanine (from green tea), hops extract, passion flower extract, chamomile extract, lemon balm extract, and melatonin. Do they work? It's hard to say. You can purchase each of these substances individually and test them. At the same time, the 3 mg of melatonin in some combination may be enough to produce sleep. If remedies like these herbal combinations do not work, consider other types of natural combinations, but also consider higher doses of melatonin.

Other natural remedies that can also help promote sleep include *L-Trytophan* or *5-HTP.* These amino acids often cause sedation and are precursors of serotonin. They are also used for their mild antidepressant effects. Starting dosage of tryptophan is usually 500 mg but can be increased to as much as 3,000 mg. For 5-HTP, start at 50 mg, and you may increase it to as much as 500 mg. GABA is another natural supplement that is used to treat anxiety and insomnia. Ask your healthcare provider about these supplements.

Some sleep medications can be found over-the-counter. Many of them contain first-generation antihistamines, which are sedating. The most commonly used OTC medication for sleep is *Benadryl* (diphenydramine), which works well for some people. Oddly, some daytime allergy remedies contain this sedating medication, too. In a March 2000 study in the *Annals of Internal Medicine,* driving abilities were tested in people after taking the over-the-counter Benadryl, prescription Allegra (cetirizine, a non-sedating antihistamine), alcohol, or a placebo. Not surprisingly, alcohol level at a blood concentration of 0.1 percent, equal to or above legal intoxication in many places, impaired driving ability. But over-the-counter Benadryl, as the researchers wrote, "had a greater impact on driving than alcohol did."

Prescription Drugs for Sleep

What about prescription drugs specifically prescribed to promote sleep? *Ambien* (zolpiden) has been reported to cause sleepwalking in some people. This dangerous tendency has been seen before in earlier sleep medications. Many stories about dangerous sleep walking, as well as amnesia while driving, working, and traveling by air or train, emerged in the 1980s and 1990s with a top-selling sleep remedy, Halcion (triaozolam). With these widely publicized side effects, the real shock was that the FDA hasn't required adequate testing of this possibility with newer sleep remedies like Ambien.

If you need prescription medication for insomnia, work closely with your doctor to use it selectively and only as needed so that you do not develop problems or become dependent on it. Also, ask your doctor about muscle relaxants and whether they might reduce your muscle tightness or tendon pain. These types of drugs may enhance your ability to sleep

The Surprising Value
of Doing Your Own Research

In 2013, Donna E. sent a large packet of information to me. I read it and felt it was important. I asked for Donna's permission to include some of it in the book, and she kindly consented.

Donna explained to me:

> I am a year and two months from a severe Cipro reaction, and considering the fact that my joints virtually fell apart, I am able to function fairly well. In May 2012, I was given Cipro for a bladder infection, and yes, 1,000 mg IV of prednisone, too. The next day every joint in my body became inflamed. I got searing pain everywhere. I just wanted to die. I cried all of the time. My thyroid swelled and I couldn't swallow. I had heart arrhythmias and pain in my eyes.

Donna's doctor gave her alpha lipoic acid infusions, which provided her only some benefit. Her doctor then recommended vitamin C infusions, but this created crystals and bleeding in her urine. Eventually, she learned that Cipro damaged the mitochondrial membranes of cells, producing oxidative stress, which was worsened by the calcium oxalate crystals caused by the vitamin C infusions. Donna began reading and learning. She discovered that oxalates could cause tissue injury and impair her ability to heal. Oxalates can get into heart muscle, joints, nerves, thyroid, and also cross the blood brain barrier. They can also become deposited in many muscles and cause painful movement. Donna then requested a urine test for calcium oxalates from her doctor. It was positive.

According to Donna, "I wondered where the calcium oxalate was coming from. I ate a healthy diet, yet even foods such as nuts, spinach, soy, and chocolate can be quite high in oxalates. I went on a low-oxalate diet and started the gradual, eight-month process of dumping oxalates. This treatment had the most dramatic effect on how I felt. As the oxalates left my body, things started to get better and have continued to improve." It became clear to me that an approach with this effect would be a welcome turnaround to many people with FTS. I encouraged Donna to speak with people who have established websites on FTS and the destructive effects the drugs can cause. Donna's knowledge has helped to provide a lot of benefit to many people.

Donna continues to learn and inform people about oxalates. She wrote to me:

> Oxalates are substances that are normal byproducts of the cellular metabolism of foods. However, with high intake of foods that produce oxalates, or in people prone to producing high levels of oxalates due to their metabolism, problems can occur. Best known are kidney stones. Foods high in oxalates include some cereals, nuts, mustard greens, collards, okra, spinach, potatoes and sweet potatoes, tomatoes, beans, apricots, figs, kiwi, whole wheat, barley, and soy.

Donna has showed me pages and pages, and chapters and chapters, of foods rich in oxalates, diets safe for people sensitive to oxalates, and the body's metabolic mechanisms. She has done her homework. I congratulated Donna for the high quality of her work that has provided her with substantial relief from her FTS, especially because she'd been given both Cipro and steroids. Her experience with an oxalate free-diet sounded plausible to me and worthy of further investigation.

I referred Donna to several of the websites that have dedicated their work to helping inform people about FTS and providing others with information that might help them move forward. I have encouraged her to do the same, and report on the responses of her approach to others. I hope Donna gets to share her findings online for others to see and hopefully benefit from as well. When I think about the many doctors who are so quick to dismiss the research of people, I marvel at Donna and people like her who have so worked hard to inform themselves and many others with FTS.

without resorting to sleep medications. One of my first patients with FTS slept well with a modest dose of nightly Valium, because it provided her with excellent muscle relaxation. Remember, different individuals respond differently to different medications even at the same doses. Work closely with a doctor with a good knowledge of the various older and newer sleep remedies.

CHRONIC FATIGUE WITH FTS

Chronic musculoskeletal or neurological pain, cardiac or gastrointestinal systems, brain fog, poor sleep, bad dreams, chronic anxiety or depression, as well as the inability to work, exercise or undertake normal everyday activities—all of these may contribute to the chronic fatigue that sometimes accompanies FTS. The substances listed here are thought to help fatigue syndromes. Whether these substances are effective for the fatigue with FTS is unknown. If possible, work with doctors who have treated people with FTS or who have at least heard about it. They may be hard to find. If you prefer alternative therapies instead of drugs, find a provider with experience with alternative and complementary therapies, hopefully someone with knowledge of the supplements mentioned in this book. Here are some possibilities for FTS with significant chronic fatigue.

Coenzyme Q10 and Pyrroloquinolone Quinone (PQQ)

Most people have heard of *coenzyme Q10* (CoQ10), a supplement that boosts the capability of cells to generate energy. CoQ10 was introduced in the early 1980s at a low dosage of 10 mg three times a day. Over the years, alternative doctors found that higher doses provide better results. Many believe that fatigue syndromes are a manifestation of mitochondrial failure. CoQ10 helps in the transformation of fats and sugars into energy, which in turn restores mitochondrial functioning and has a beneficial effect on overall health, especially on cardiac and brain function. Absorption is improved when CoQ10 is taken with a meal containing oil or fat, or simply a teaspoon of olive oil.

Pyrroloquinolone Quinone, or PQQ, is another coenzyme and micronutrient that provides further defense against mitochondrial delay. In addition, it stimulates growth of fresh mitochondria. In doing so, it reduces the risk of degenerative disease in the brain, heart, and muscles by providing these structures with enhanced antioxidant protection.

D-Ribose

Another supplement that you might research for fatigue is D-ribose. D-ribose is a five-carbon monosaccharide that is produced in all living cells. It forms part of the carbohydrate aspect of DNA and RNA. D-ribose is also involved in the cellular process necessary for the production of ATP. In 2006, a research article in the *Journal of Alternative and Complementary Medicine* noted, "fibromyalgia (FM) and chronic fatigue syndrome (CFS) are debilitating syndromes that are often associated with impaired cellular energy metabolism.

As D-ribose has been shown to increase cellular energy synthesis in heart and skeletal muscle," the researchers undertook a pilot study to evaluate if D-ribose could improve the symptoms of these conditions in patients. The study included forty-one patients with FM and/or CFS. The D-ribose was well-tolerated and produced improvement in all five scales: energy, sleep, mental clarity, pain intensity, and well-being. Approximately 66 percent of subjects experienced significant improvement while on D-ribose. Alternative health expert Andrew Weil, M.D., has also noted that D-ribose may reduce the pain and fatigue of patients with fibromyalgia and chronic fatigue syndrome.

S-Adenoysl-L-Methionine (SAMe)

Discovered in 1952, SAMe is formed naturally in the human body from the amino acid methionine in action with ATP. SAMe has been available in the United States as a dietary supplement since 1999 and has been available in some European countries one or two decades earlier. Discovered by accident to be helpful for osteoarthritis (the arthritis of injury or aging), SAMe is also used for heart disease, fibromyalgia, bursitis, tendinitis, and chronic lower back pain.

SAMe effectiveness has also been used for depression. SAMe can increase the neurotransmitter dopamine in the brain, acting similarly to the antidepressant Wellbutrin (bupropion). Both substances can exert a caffeine-like clinical effect that some people find energizing and therefore helpful for fatigue conditions. Others, however, may find this energizing effect to be anxiety-provoking. Like Wellbutrin, SAMe does not cause the sexual dysfunctions frequently seen with SSRI types of antidepressants, such as Prozac, Lexapro, and Zoloft, or with SNRI antidepressants, such as Effexor and Cymbalta. The prescription drug Wellbutrin also is occasionally beneficial for fatigue. The usual recommended starting dose is 150 mg; however, many people do well with Wellbutrin when started lower at 75 mg daily, or even lower by splitting the tablets, especially if you are sensitive to activating substances like coffee.

Medical Stimulants

For a person who is severely fatigued for a long time, I would discuss the possibility of an amphetamine-type medication such as the drug *Provigil* (modafinil). This drug, as well as its newest version, *Nuvigil,* are approved for treating narcolepsy. They are listed as stimulants. Find a doctor who is experienced with this type of medication and who knows how to use it carefully. As you improve, you may be able to gradually reduce your dosage and gradually discontinue. First, have your doctor check for any condition that may cause severe lethargy, such as hypothyroidism, malnutrition, or adrenal fatigue.

I rarely prescribe these drugs. But one patient who had been chronically depressed with serious fatigue for years (not the result of FTS) responded well to the antidepressant Cymbalta (duloxetine), although her fatigue did not budge. While in Mexico, her family doctor prescribed Provigil and her fatigue improved substantially. I continued the regimen for her, and her improvement endured for several years without the development of tolerance to the drug. This approach should be done carefully, with frequent follow-up visits, with a doctor knowledgeable about these types of medications.

CONCLUSION

As many of you have encountered, many doctors are not pleased or are downright skeptical about information you have discovered about your FTS, especially if you found some of it on the internet. Some doctors seem to take it almost personally if you made the diagnosis of FTS from things you have read yourself or heard from others. But if you have no other recourse, what do doctors expect you to do? Nothing? I believe that humans are built to search and learn and pursue ideas. I encourage you to use any means available for you to identify the source of your condition and the treatments that might benefit you. No one is more motivated to learn about and understand your FTS than you.

Over the years, I have spoken with many people whose lives have been stricken by reactions to FQs. These reactions can differ considerably from person to person. One man wrote to me of doing very well on the paleo diet. Why not consider all of the possibilities, as long as it is done safely? Communicate with your doctors or other healthcare professionals, integrative specialists, herbalists, etc. Interact with other individuals who have been injured or disabled by FQs. View the websites that have been established and learn what is worthwhile from those that offer useful information. You should consider any information that may be helpful, relevant, or important in diagnosing this very serious and often long-lasting medical problem. For many years I have been impressed by the community that has grown from the tens of thousands who have experienced FTS. Much of what this book contains could never have been written without the efforts of the "floxed" community and the healthcare professionals who have sought to understand FTS and help heal those with it.

9

What We Must Do Now

The past few chapters in Part 2 covered many aspects of fluoroquinolone toxicity syndrome and various medical therapies and alternative approaches that people have tested or are considering for their FTS. Some people have been quite resourceful in the methods they have tried while seeking to understand and improve their conditions. Yet many thousands have not found solutions for their pain.

I propose the following four action steps in order to stop fluoroquinolone toxicity in its tracks. These steps will not only help those who are currently affected by FTS, but also take measures to prevent fluoroquinolones from claiming any more victims going forward. In addition, these action steps will strive towards precluding similar catastrophes with other medications in the future.

ACTION ONE
An Initiative Involving the Entire Medical System

Clearly, there is much more we must do about FTS. Every aspect of the medical system must be directly involved in solving the problem. Cipro was approved in the late 1980s, almost thirty years ago, and we have yet to make any major progress in dealing with FTS, even with the newer FQs, such as Levaquin, which was approved a decade later.

The FDA has continued to increase and strengthen the warnings on the six FQs, but we learned long ago that FDA warnings are often not very effective. Every few years, another black-box label has been sent directly to doctors, yet the number of reports to the FDA keep on climbing, now topping 50,000 individual cases of serious FTS. And the FDA now adds that FTS can be permanent in some people. What a chilling admission! This cannot continue.

The FDA still claims that people at risk of FTS are mainly seniors, mostly over sixty. This has been dead wrong for two decades! The FDA's own data show that more than 55 percent of FQ cases are people in their fifties or younger, and frequently involve children, athletes, and young women prone to urinary problems—who often do not need FQs but receive them anyway!

ACTION TWO
A Simple, Rapid Test to Diagnose FTS

Doctors and patients alike will breathe a deep sigh of relief when we are able to summon their abilities to identify FTS in a patient, just like we have done with rapid office test for strep throat infections. It is very difficult for doctors to accurately diagnose many conditions without proper testing. This is especially true for FTS, which can impact so many different systems (musculoskeletal, neurological, skin, cardiac, gastro-intestinal, rheumatologic, etc.) and to such varying degrees of injury. We don't need the sophisticated testing done by Dr. Joe King and his group (Chapter 5). We don't need slow and expensive DNA testing at the outset. We just need a test that can give us a diagnosis with which doctors can work.

A few years ago, I was involved in the case of Monica Molloy, a young, athletic teacher who developed severe tendon and joint injuries that have handicapped her from her work as a gym teacher for five years and ongoing. She had been having mild pain in her lower abdomen. At a nearby minute clinic, she displayed no signs of a bladder infection or appendicitis, but the doctor strongly recommended she go to the local hospital ER for tests to rule out an ectopic pregnancy. She and her husband had been trying to get pregnant, so she followed the recommendation although she felt fine and had no symptoms of illness. The ER tests were normal, yet the ER doctor insisted Monica take the Cipro he prescribed "in order to be safe," as she testified in court. In other words, he scared her into taking the drug (which she did not need!) Five days later, she developed acute symptoms of head and neck aches, and diverse tendon pain. She stopped the Cipro, and has been ill ever since.

At the trial, the doctor claimed Monica had a kidney infection and had needed treatment with a strong antibiotic like Cipro, yet the doctor did not indicate any sign of kidney or any other infection in his notes. The Mayo Clinic lists five cardinal signs of a kidney infection: fever, back or flank pain, urge to urinate, burning sensation or pain with urination, and blood or pus in the urine. Monica had absolutely none of these symptoms and had been fine all day long. Besides, she had only come to the ER to rule out a possible ectopic pregnancy, which the tests showed she did not have. Two days after starting her Cipro, her urine culture came back normal. There was no sign of infection and never was.

My sense upon reading the ER notes was that the doctor did a very cursory evaluation of Monica and prescribed her the Cipro on autopilot, like many doctors do in a hectic emergency room. Doctors in the ER are very busy, often taking care of multiple patients at the same time, and can sometimes even mix some patients' cases up in their haste. Besides, hadn't they been told over and over that these FQs were eminently safe?

Certainly there was nothing whatsoever in Monica's history or excellent physical condition for the ER doctor to prescribe her such a highly potent antibiotic, yet doctors have become accustomed to prescribing FQs for many symptoms, including mild ones. Or nonexistent ones. In addition, this doctor found many other doctors to back up his use of Cipro, many of whom were members of an ER doctors' association. Monica's attorney found others to rebut them, but overall it was a tough case to win because there are no tests to prove that Monica's injuries were caused by the Cipro. In fact, many FQ injuries are difficult to prove because tests are usually normal. It is hard to convince a jury unless you have an injury like an Achilles tendon rupture, which is demonstrated on MRI. Monica, like many with FTS, has pain in many areas, but diverse tendon injury is not demonstrable.

Unless we have a simple, rapid test that can show FTS, FQs will continue to be prescribed unnecessarily for tens of millions of patients each year. Doctors will continue to fail to properly diagnose FTS, and injured patients will not get properly diagnosed and treated, or have their proper day in court.

ACTION THREE
Create a National Medication Safety Board

I called for the creation of a National Medication Safety Board back in 2001, when medications killed 104,000 Americans and hospitalized 2 million *every year*. Prescription medications were the fourth leading cause of death in the United States annually. Things are no better now, plus we have the Cipro catastrophe, going on for nearly thirty years. We need a better system! So have said many of the top pharmacologists in the medical field, including Drs. Carl Peck, Raymond Woosley, Jerry Avorn, and many other highly admired leaders.

The responsibilities and duties of my proposed National Medical Safety Board would entail the following:

1. Monitor new drugs as soon as they are approved in order to promptly confirm they are safe and effective.

2. Quickly review all safety information from drug companies, the National Institutes of Health, and independent and other sources. These agencies would immediately notify the NMSB of any newly discovered drug toxicities.

3. With each new drug, develop a centralized database that incorporates new safety information. This current and comprehensive information would be accessible to the health community and to the public, and NMSB may encourage public disclosure when necessary.

4. Provide ongoing scrutiny of drug reaction reports, using computer analyses to quickly identify trends.

5. When safety issues arrive, hold public hearing with representatives of the FDA, drug companies, doctors, consumers, etc.

6. Quickly recommend and mobilize actions necessary to maximize drug safety and minimize FQ risks.

7. Take actions necessary for improving doctors' knowledge and methods when choosing to prescribe potentially toxic medications like FQs.

8. Ensure that doctors are fully informed about safety risks with FQs and when the drugs might and might not be used. Doctors must be educated that FQs are not first-line drugs for mild infections, despite what drug company studies, advertising, or reps claim.

9. Hold doctors accountable to ensuring that patients are fully informed of serious FQ risks.

10. Ensure that drug companies provide annual, comprehensive updates on FQs. This would guarantee a current and accurate source of information.

ACTION FOUR
Develop Treatment Methods that Work

This would be the primary directive of the NMSB. For now, it must also become the primary goal for the FDA, the drug industry, medical societies, and all medical practitioners. As I've said previously, I've spoken to approximately 500 people, just a small sample of the many thousands of people chronically injured by FTS who are still reading, looking around, seeing doctors, and hoping to find answers. And now I believe we may have some answers. They are not complete answers, but they have helped a lot of people. Meanwhile, the NMSB would lead us much further and help people much more quickly and fully.

TREATMENT RESEARCH POSSIBILITES

In Chapter 6, I described a series of studies conducted over the span of a decade. These revealing studies clearly indicated the destructive impact of Cipro on musculoskeletal structures when given to young rats. The injuries were massive. FQs impair magnesium metabolism in cells, thereby causing injury in many types of tissues, including musculoskeletal tissues. Injuries from impaired magnesium metabolism can also make nerve cells a favorite FQ target. FQs can also block tissue repair cells injured from magnesium depletion, which explains why the injuries from FQs may last so long.

In the next phase of the study in rats, magnesium was added to their feed. After several days on the magnesium-rich diet, the rats were given a dosage of Cipro, the same amount as the earlier group of rats. But the amount of injuries from Cipro was much less, and the ability of the magnesium to block the injuries was extraordinary, reducing the injury rate by more than 80 percent overall!

This is a promising point to initiate research into preventing and treating FTS. One problem is that we must remember that magnesium also inactivates FQs and therefore cannot be given simultaneously with these antibiotics, or they will lose their antibacterial effectiveness. So how can the beneficial effect of magnesium be used without inactivating the FQs? Studies have already shown that people can take a FQ, and in four to six hours take antacids without inactivating the antibiotics. So one obvious study should give a FQ to the animals, then give magnesium four to six hours later. Will the FQ still work, and will the magnesium still block most injuries? These are important questions with important implications.

This research can proceed in several other directions, too. First and foremost, the testing of FQs must start at discovering ways to prevent the occurrence of FTS. For example, we can test several types of FQs in rats and other animals, and then we can test the FQs with several types, doses, and frequencies of magnesium. Which forms of FQs and magnesium work best together? This line of research may lead us to FQs that work better and more safely than any before. And FTS may become rare or better yet, perhaps it may make FQ reactions ancient history.

And what about those people already afflicted with FTS? It is one thing to prevent an adverse reaction, but something entirely different to reverse a condition that has already occurred. And it is altogether a different thing to stop a problem that is still evolving versus reversing a problem with tissue damage that has already existed for months or years. Or reversing a condition such as tendinitis with limited damage and pain versus reversing a tendon rupture with severe pain and major mechanical damage. This is why we need a National Medication Safety Board: to organize and spearhead such complicated, diverse, and important undertakings.

OTHER ESSENTIAL TRACTS OF RESEARCH

Are there other substances that might augment or work better than magnesium? There are many tracks that can and must be followed. We already know that zinc, tested in rats, sometimes reverses injuries from Cipro. Surely this mineral needs to be examined closely as soon as possible. Could it provide greater benefits than magnesium, or possibly multiply the benefits by using zinc with magnesium? Might others also play a useful protective role?

Studies have also shown significantly reduced FQ-induced injuries with the use of vitamin E, a potent antioxidant. Are there any other antioxidants that might help further reduce injuries from FQs? Remember, FTS is caused in part from severe oxidative stress to the tissue of bacteria, animals, and humans. Might other antioxidants add greater protection from FQ damage? Might there be a specific cocktail of substances that might provide the best antioxidant protection?

We know that N-acetylcysteine (NAC) also reduces injuries caused by FQs. This natural substance has already been widely tested in emergency rooms for decades for its use in Tylenol overdose and in doctors' offices for other health purposes. More study must be done on this well-proven substance. I've already said that the standard dosage of NAC is 600 mg three times daily. Yet Dr. Alan Gaby, M.D., past president of the American Holistic Medical Association and a longtime colleague, states that for some psychiatric conditions, up to 2,400 mg a day is used. Would this dose be safe and even more effective in people with FTS? And would an even higher intravenous dosage of NAC help even more? All of this must be sorted out in research centers.

Or we might consider adding NAC and some of the other substances mentioned above to a standard cocktail when FQ reactions occur in people. Remember in Chapter 6, the early, severe FTS reaction in Sean was halted by about two-thirds within hours after he was given an intravenous infusion of magnesium. He continued taking oral magnesium and other supplements, and he gradually returned to health within a few more weeks. Sean thought he was having a vicious migraine attack. So did his doctor. It didn't matter that they were wrong about the problem. With the magnesium, they had the right solution.

CONCLUSION

There might be dozens of other safe substances that might guarantee even greater protection from FQ toxicity reactions. This might allow people to use FQs carefully for some serious infections. These answers seem quite possible if we undertake serious, broad studies, led by a serious and determined and properly funded agency: the National Medication Safety Board. We are well overdue, and the need is greater than ever. We have hundreds of thousands of people with chronic, painful, and disabling FTS. The time is now.

Conclusion

Many people with FTS have said to me, "I never imagined an antibiotic could cause so much injury to people." Antibiotics have a noble history spanning nearly a hundred years of protecting people from infections and death. Terrible scourges that packed hospitals for many decades during the twentieth century virtually disappeared before the twenty-first. The question about antibiotics has always been, "Are they strong enough to do the job?" This explains why doctors often start patients on antibiotics for a suspected urinary tract infection even before the tests have been proven positive. This is why some patients are prescribed 500 mg twice daily of Cipro, even though it has not been proven that even 250 mg is essential.

Doctors have to worry that using a low dose of an antibiotic, antifungal, or anticancer drug can be more harmful than using a high dose. A UTI can turn into a kidney infection, that can turn into a blood infection, that can lead to death. Concerns like these are often in a doctor's mind when dealing with an infectious disease. This is why it is so important that the early research on antibiotics, such as on FQs, has been thorough. Once a new antibiotic has been researched for use by doctors and released into public use by a drug manufacturer, it is difficult to catch up. Even now, thirty years later, the FDA is still trying to alert the healthcare community of the clear benefits and serious risks of FQs.

CRIES FOR HELP

The number of cases of fluoroquinolone toxicity syndrome reported to the FDA by mid-February 2014 was around 50,000. The number is not exact, and here's why. Working with the reports submitted to the FDA takes some thought. For instance, there is an important difference between the terms *cases* and *reports*. The sheer number of reports sent to the FDA can exaggerate the number of actual cases, or incidents, that have occurred. This is because reports may arrive from more than one source: patients, doctors, pharmacists, drug companies. Thus, several reports may be submitted regarding the same case. To avoid counting these redundant reports, we designed our search of FDA records to wean out the duplicates and provide us with a reliable number of actual cases, or incidents, of FQ toxicity reactions.

In January 2014, with the help of Paul Danese of FDAble.com, a company that obtains FDA records and conducts streamlined searches, we undertook a rigorous analysis of the records. We also dismissed cases in which a FQ was listed as a secondary cause, that is, one of several possible causes that could include other drugs or illnesses. Instead, we selected only those cases in which the FQ was the primary and therefore most probable cause of injury—so probable that it would be accepted as proof in a court of law.

Our research determined that during the fifteen-year span beginning in the fourth quarter of 1997 to the fourth quarter of 2012, 41,290 individual cases of FQ toxicity were reported to the FDA. This amounts to about 2,950 cases a year. Using this number, we can generally estimate that by the end of 2013, approximately 45,000 cases of FTS had been reported to the FDA. And by the last quarter of 2015, about 50,000. But as I have said previously, RxISK.org has counted far larger numbers.

Nor do the FDA's numbers include the ten years of FQ injuries that occurred from 1988, when Cipro was approved, through the first three quarters of 1998. The numbers during this ten-year span are difficult to estimate since other FQs entered the market and some were removed because of dangerous side effects or poor sales. For this reason, let's just stick with the likely number of 50,000 cases of FTS reported to the FDA by the end of 2015, although we know that the numbers reported to the FDA are likely gross underestimates.

The Tip of the Iceberg

If 50,000 is the estimated number of FQ injuries reported to the FDA from the fourth quarter of 1997 until the end of 2015, then this equals an average of about 2,950 cases per year. When you consider that FQs are prescribed around 30 million times annually, a few thousand cases of serious side effects per year may not seem too bad.

However, we must consider two additional factors. First, many FQ toxicities are extremely severe. Other antibiotics can cause severe reactions such as liver failure or disfiguring skin reactions, but they are very rare. Serious, disabling FQ toxic reactions are not so rare, and they are often very severe. Second and most important, the 50,000 cases reported to the FDA are almost certainly a gross underestimate of the problem. In prior studies, experts have repeatedly found that the number of cases of medication reactions reported to the FDA represents only the tip of the iceberg. Only about 2 to 5 percent of adverse drug reactions from medications are reported to the FDA. Indeed, in one large study, the percentage of reactions reported to the FDA was less than even one percent. Some of these statistics were determined in studies undertaken by the FDA itself.

Let's assume that a higher number such as 5 percent of FTS cases have been reported to the FDA. Then we must multiply the 50,000 FDA cases by a factor of twenty to get a full picture. This amounts to one million cases of FTS, more than 55,000 a year. Even for drugs prescribed millions of times annually, this is a frighteningly high number.

LOOKING TO THE FUTURE

I want to emphasize this: FQs are important medications. They save lives. We need FQs—to be used properly, cautiously, and intelligently. FQs are too valuable and too powerful to be controlled by drug companies seeking to make a profit. Our economic system has its benefits and weaknesses. Once a drug is discovered to have serious dangers, it no longer should be kept in the hands of profit-driven entities. That is why we must have something like the National Medication Safety Board I proposed in Chapter 9 step in—a neutral party to take charge and run this important undertaking.

Remember, after a major airplane crash, the government doesn't call the FAA (Federal Aviation Administration), which mainly helps regulate airplane commerce. And it doesn't call in airplane groups involved in recreation or sales. The government calls the National Transportation Safety Board (NTSB). This is the agency responsible for examining the airplane disaster, for analyzing the findings, and for recommending beneficial changes to improve air travel safety. The NTSB is the big gun when major airline accidents occur.

Well, major problems are occurring in many of the 30 million people who take FQs each year in the United States and many millions of others elsewhere. We must quickly create a National Medication Safety Board, or certainly a much stronger and more forceful FDA, because the FQ problem has extended way too far and for far too long. The problem is way beyond the capability of the current FDA and drug industry. We need an NMSB or similar agency with true federal powers so it can lead and coordinate the drug companies, Centers for Disease Control, Institutes of Health, as well as major medical research centers and major treatment centers. There is so much we must learn and do. We must identify and correct the problems, and we must do so quickly!

Everyone must pitch in to end this scourge of FTS, which threatens every person, every family, and every group everywhere. Progress has been woefully slow. Cipro first appeared commercially in 1988, and reports of major nerve damage and tendon ruptures, etc., began years earlier. Now, thirty years later, we must move farther and faster to halt the FTS catastrophe. We need more exposure and dissemination of the problem, as by Jane Brody in the *New York Times* in 2012, and by Idelle Davidson in the *Washington Post* in August 2015, and with a growing number of recent reports by others. We need much more exposure to the public about the problem. We still have a very long way to go.

I never imagined the problem of fluoroquinolone toxicity would grow into a national disaster. My hope now is that this book has shed some much-needed light on FTS, and that now that we have fully identified many of the problems, we can move forward forcefully and effectively, and do something meaningful and hopeful. That is my hope. In my view, this book is woefully insufficient on several levels. It contains only what I have seen or heard, or read or thought. I have been very determined to get the word out as I did fifteen years ago, and to encourage the healthcare system to pay attention to these people and their families, and to proceed with the work that is required of us. I believe that we can solve the problems with fluoroquinolone antibiotics with better and smarter use; by becoming more knowledgeable about how FQs injure people; and by finding therapies like magnesium and NAC and hopefully many more that allow us to use these antibiotics safely.

When I first became a doctor at age twenty-five, I really did not know why. It was my parents' dream, not my own. For me, medicine was an odyssey that took me to many arenas and finally delivered me at age forty-nine to my place in pharmacology, where I love to research and read and learn and write. As I said in the beginning, this book has its flaws, but my hope is that it has delivered its message, and that it will lead to a better, safer, healthier place for all of those I had the privilege to speak and work with over the years.

I wish the best to all of you. My great hope is that we can solve the fluoroquinolone toxicity problem quickly and fully, and that you, too, can start returning to a more normal life again.

Glossary

This book occasionally uses scientific and medical terms that are common in discussions about fluoroquinolones and fluoroquinolone toxicity syndrome, but may not be completely familiar to you. You may also hear these terms when working with doctors and other healthcare specialists. To help you better understand fluoroquinolones and FTS and participate in discussions with your physician, definitions are provided below.

Achilles tendon. The largest tendon in the body. It connects the heel to the calf, stretching from the back of the ankle up to the calf muscles.

Arthropathy. A disease of the joints.

Bacteriocidal. A substance or drug that kills bacteria.

Bacteriostatic. A substance or drug that prevents the growth of bacteria.

Cardiac arrhythmia. An abnormal heart beat—either too fast, too slow, or erratic. Cardiac arrhythmias can result in palpitations, lightheadedness, shortness of breath, and chest pain.

Cardiovascular. Relating to the heart and blood vessels.

Central nervous system (CNS). The part of the nervous system that comprises the brain and the spinal cord. The CNS coordinates the activity of the entire nervous system and controls thought processes, conducts movement, and register sensations throughout the body.

Chelate complexes. Complex compounds consisting of a central metal atom attached to a large molecule.

Chelation. The bonding of ions and molecules to metal ions.

Chrondrotoxic. Toxic to cartilage.

Contraindication. A condition or factor that indicates against the advisability of an otherwise typical remedy or treatment due to the harm it would cause the patient. For example, certain medications are fine to take on their own but *contraindicated* for simultaneous use due to adverse drug reactions, such as warfarin, a blood thinner used to treat blood clots, and aspirin.

DNA-adduct. A segment of DNA bound to a cancer-causing chemical.

Electromyography (EMG). A medicinal technique used to assess the health of skeletal muscles and motor neurons, or the nerve cells that control them.

Floxed. A term that is sometimes used by individuals affected with fluoroquinolone toxicity syndrome, referring to the damage fluoroquinolones have done to their bodies. The "floxed" community often refer to themselves as "floxies."

Fluoroquinolone Antibiotics. Quinolone antibiotics which contain a fluorine atom in their chemical structure.

Gastrointestinal. Relating to the stomach and the intestines.

Intestinal flora. The *symbiotic* (mutually beneficial) bacteria naturally occurring in the intestine.

Malaise. A general feeling of illness, discomfort, or uneasiness, the exact cause of which is unsure.

Musculoskeletal. Relating to or involving both the muscles and the bones.

Myalgia. Pain in a muscle or group of muscles.

Myasthenia gravis. A condition causing abnormal weakness or fatigue in the muscles.

Myopathy. A clinical disorder of the skeletal muscles.

Norepinephrine reuptake inhibitor. A type of drug that acts as a reuptake inhibitor for the neurotransmitters norepinephrine, or noradrenaline, and epinephrine, or adrenaline.

Opiod analgesic. Pain relievers that act on the central nervous system. They are typically prescribed for moderate to severe pain.

Oxalate. A salt or ester of oxalic acid, an organic compound that commonly occurs in many plants and vegetables.

Peripheral nervous system. The second part of the nervous system, which consists of the nerves and *ganglia* (nerve cell clusters) outside the brain and spinal cord. The PNS functions to connect the CNS to the limbs and organs, connecting the brain and spinal cord to the rest of the body.

Peripheral neuropathy. Damage to or disease affecting the nerves. Peripheral neuropathies can impair sensations, movement, gland or organ function. Often, peripheral neuropathies cause weakness, numbness and pain in the hands and feet.

Pharmacovigilance. The pharmacological science relating to drug safety, in particular the detection, assessment, monitoring and prevention of the adverse effects of pharmaceutical drugs.

Psychosis. A mental disorder characterized by a disconnection from reality.

Psychosomatic. A physical illness or other condition relating to the interaction of the mind and body. Psychosomatic disorders cause physical symptoms but are thought to be caused by emotional and psychological stress.

Quinolones. A class of broad-spectrum, bactericidal antibiotics.

Raynaud's disease. Also referred to as Reynaud's phenomenon, a condition in which some areas of the body feel numb and cool in certain circumstances.

Reactive oxygen species (ROS). Free radicals, a type of unstable molecule that easily reacts with other molecules in a cell. A build up of ROS in cells can potentially cause damage to DNA, RNA, and proteins.

Rhabdomyolysis. A breakdown of muscle tissue that releases a damaging protein in the blood.

Tendinitis. Inflammation of the tendons.

Tendinopathy. A disease of the tendon.

Somnolence. Sleepiness; a state of drowsiness.

References

Open Letter to the Senate Committee on Health, Education & Labor

1. Adikwu, E, Brambaifa, N. "Ciprofloxacin induced in chrondotoxicity and tendinopathy." *American Journal of Pharmacology and Toxicology* 2012; 7(3)94-100.

2. Biundo, JJ Jr, Mipro, RJ Jr, Fahey, P. "Sports related and other soft tissue injuries, tendinitis, bursitis, and occupation-related syndromes." *Current Opinion in Rheumatology* 1997; 9(3)151-154.

3. Cohen, JS, "Peripheral Neuropathy Associated with Fluoroquinolone Antibiotics." *Annals of Pharmacotherapy* 2001; 35(12): 1540-1547.

4. Corps, AN, Harrall , RL, Curry, VA, et al. "Ciprofloxacin enhances the stimulation of matrix metalloproteinase 3 expression by interleukin-1beta in human tendon derived cells: a potential mechanism of fluoroquinolone induced tendinopathy." *Arthritis and Rheumatism* 2002, 46(11):3039-3040.

5. Gürbay, A, Gonthier, B, Signorini-Allibe, N, Barret, L, Favier, A, and Hincal, F. "Ciprofloxacin-induced DNA damage in Primary Culture of Rat Astrocytes and Protection by Vitamin E." *Neurotoxicology* 2006; 27(1):6-10.

6. Hall, MM, Finnoff, JT, Smith, J. "Musculoskeletal Complications of Fluoroquinolones: Guidelines and Precautions for Usage in the Athletic Population." *Physical Medicine and Rehabilitation* 2011; 3(2):132-142.

7. Kaleagasioglu, E, Olcay, E. "Fluoroquinolone-induced tendinopathy: Etiology and Preventative Measures." *Tohoku Journal of Experimental Medicine* 2005; 226:251-258.

8. Khaliq, Y, Zhanel, GG. "Musculoskeletal Injury Associated with Fluoroquinolone Antibiotics." *Clinical Plastic Surgery* 2005; 32(4):495-50.

9. Kim, GK, Del Rosso, JQ. "The Risk of Fluoroquinolone-Induced Tendinopathy and Tendon Rupture: What Does the Clinician Need to Know?" *Journal of Clinical and Aesthetic Dermatology* 2010; 3(41):49-54.

10. Melhus, A. "Fluoroquinolones and Tendon Disorders." *Expert Opinion on Drug Safety* 2005; 4(2):299-309.

11. Pouzaud, F, Thevenin, K, Warnet, JM et al. "In Vitro Disinhibituion of Fluoro-

quinolones: Toxicity on Tendon Cells: Involvement of Oxidative Stress." *Journal of Pharmacology and Experimental Therapeutics* 2003; 308(1):394-402.

12. Shakibaei, M, de Souza, P, van Sickle, D, Stahlmann, R. "Biochemical Changes in Achilles Tendon from Juvenile Dogs After Treatment with Ciprofloxacin or Feeding a Magnesium Deficient Diet." *Archives of Toxicology* 2001; 75(6):369-374.

13. Tsai, WC, Yang, YM. "Fluoroquinolone Associated Tendinopathy." *Chang Gung Medical Journal* 2011; 24(5):461-467.

14. Williams, RJ, Attia, E, Wickiewicz, TL, Hannafin, JA. "The Effect of Metabolism." *American Journal of Sports Medicine* 2000; 28(3):364-369.

Chapter 1. The Most Popular Antibiotic in America

1. Cohen, JS, "Peripheral Neuropathy Associated with Fluoroquinolone Antibiotics." *Annals of Pharmacotherpay* 2001; 35(12):1540-47.

2. Bailey, RR, Natale, R, Linton, AL. "Nalidixic Acid Arthralgia." *Canadian Medical Association Journal* 1972; 107(7):604-5.

3. Bailey, RR, Kirk, JA, Peddie, BA. "Norfloxacin-induced rheumatic disease." *New Zealand Medical Journal* 1983; 96(736, July):590.

4. McEwan, SR, Davey, J. "Ciprofloxacin and tenosynovitis." *Lancet*, 1988(2):900.

5. Cohen, C. "Risk of troglitazone apparent before approval in USA." *Diabetologia*, 2006(6): 1454-1455.

6. Cohen, JS. "How Celecoxib could be safer how valdecoxib might have been." *Annals of Pharmacotherapy* 2005; 39:1542-45.

7. Cohen, JS. "Should rosuvastatin be withdrawn from the market?" *Lancet* 2004: 1579.

8. Cohen, JS. "Statins and low-density lipoprotein cholesterol levels." *American Journal of Medicine* 2003; 115(1):74-75.

9. Cohen, JS. "Why aren't lower, effective OTC doses available earlier by prescription?" *Annals of Pharmacotherapy* 2004; 38(10):1743-1746.

10. Cohen, JS. "Tablet Splitting: Imperfect Perhaps, but Better Than Excessive Dosing." *Journal of the American Pharmacy Association* 2002; 42(2):160-162.

11. Cohen, JS. "Antidepressants: An avoidable and solvable controversy." *Annals of Pharmacotherapy* 2004; 38(10):1743-1746.

12. Cohen, JS. "Clinical and ethical concerns about switching patient treatment to 'Therapeutically Interchangeable' medications." *Arch Intern Med.* 2001;161(17):2153-2154.

13. Cohen, JS. "Dose discrepancies between the Physicians' Desk Reference and the medical literature, and their possible role in the high incidence of dose-related adverse drug events." *Archives of Internal Medicine* 2001; 161:957-64.

14. Cohen, JS. "Adverse drug effects, compliance, and the initial doses of antihyper-

intensive drugs recommended by the Joint National Committee vs. the Physicians' Desk Reference." *Archives of Internal Medicine* 2001; 161:880-85.

15. Cohen, JS. "Comparison of FDA Reports of patient deaths associated with Sildenafil (Viagra) and with injectable Alprostadil (Caverject)." *Annals of Pharmacotherapy* 2001; 35:285-88.

16. Cohen, JS. "Is the product information on the Sildenafil (Viagra) adequate to facilitate optimal therapeutics and to minimize adverse events?" *Annals of Pharmacotherapy* 2001; 35:337-42.

17. Cohen, JS. "Erythromelalgia: New Theories and New Therapies." *Journal of the American Academy of Dermatology* 2000; 43:841-7.

18. Cohen, JS. "Should patients be given a low test of sildenafil (Viagra) initially?" *Drug Safety* 2000; 23:1-10.

19. Cohen, JS. "Adverse drug reactions: effective low-dose therapies for older patients." *Geriatrics;* 55(2):54-64.

20. Cohen, JS. "Preventing adverse drug reactions before they occur." Medscape Pharmacotherapy 1999; 1(2).

21. Cohen, JS. "Ways to Minimize Adverse Drug Reactions: Individualized Doses and Common Sense Are Key." *Postgraduate Medicine* 1999; 106:163-72.

22. Cohen, JS, Insel, PA. "The Physicians' Desk Reference: Problems and Possible Improvements. *Archives of Internal Medicine* 1996; 156(13):1375-80.

23. Cohen, JS. *Over Dose: The Case Against the Drug Companies. Prescription Drugs, Side Effects, and Your Health.* New York: Tarcher/Putnam, 2001.

24. Lloyd, S. "Press Release: Peripheral Neuropathy Associated with Cipro." *Annals of Pharmacotherapy* 2001. www.theannals.com.

25. Sun, LH. "Anthrax Patients' Ailments Linger." *Washington Post,* 20 April 2002, A1.

26. Benjamin M, Olmsted, M. "Anthrax Ills Mirror Cipro Side Effects." *United Press Internationa,* 15 April 2002.

27. Cohen, JS. "Open Letter to Congress on Severe, Disabling Reactions with Cipro, Levaquin, and Other Fluoroquinolone Antibiotics: Why Hasn't the FDA Acted?" www.medicationsense.com.

28. "Ben Stein's Diary." *American Spectator,* December 2001.

39. Linder JA, Stafford RS. Antibiotic Treatment of Adults with Sore Throat by Community Primary Care Physicians: A National Survey 1989-1999, Journal of the American Medical Association 2001; 286(10)1181-1186.

30. Melhus, A. "Fluoroquinolones and Tendon Disorders." *Expert Opinion on Drug Safety* 2005; 4 (2):299-309.

31. Oliphant, CM. "Quinolones: A Comprehensive Review." *American Family Physician* 2002; 65(3):455-464.

32. Avorn, J. "The Prescription as Final Common Pathway." *International Journal of Technology Assessment in Healthcare* 1995; 11(3):384-3890.

33. Ross, D, Bukata, R. "Optimizing Prescribing Practices, Part 2." *Emergency Medicine and Acute Care Essays* 1993; 17(1)15.

34. Wood, AJJ, Stein, CM, Woosley R. "Making Medicines Safer: The Need for an Independent Drug Safety Board." *New England Journal of Medicine* 1998; 339:1851-1854.

35. Bates, DW. "Drugs and Adverse Drug Reactions: How Worried Should We Be?" *Journal of the American Medical Association* 1998; 279(15):1216-17.

36. Woosley, RL. "Drug Labeling Revisions: Guaranteed to Fail?" *Journal of the American Medical Association* 2000; 284(23) 3047-3049.

37. Gilman, AG, Rall, TW, Nies, AS. *Taylor P. Goodman and Gilman's The Pharmacological Basis of Therapeutics.* New York: Pergammon Press, 1990, 1996, 2008.

38. *Drug Evaluations: Annual 1993.* Chicago: American Medical Association, 1993.

39. "Dangerous Prescription: Interview with Raymond Woosley, M.D." *Frontline,* 13 November 2013, pbs.org.

Chapter 2. Toxicity in the Tendons, Joints, and Bones

1. Lee, WT, Collins, JF. "Ciprofloxacin associated bilateral Achilles tendon rupture." Australia & *New Zealand Journal of Medicine* 1992; 5:500.

2. Ribard, P, Audisio, F. Kahn, MF, et al. "Seven Achilles tendinitis including 3 Complicated by Rupture During Fluoroquinolone Therapy," *Rheumatology* 1992: 1479-81.

3. Royer, RJ, Pierfitte, C, Netter, P. "Features of Tendon Disorders with Fluoroquinolones?" *Therapie;* 1994:75-76.

4. Huston, KA. "Achilles Tendinitis and Tendon Rupture Due to Fluoroquinolone Antibiotics." *New England Journal of Medicine* 1994; 331(11):748.

5. *Physician's Desk Reference* 1997.

6. Hall, MM, Finnoff, JT, Smith, J. "Musculoskeletal complications of fluoroquinolones: guidelines and precautions for usage in the athletic population." *Physical Medicine & Rehabilitation* 2011; 3(2):132-42.

7. *Medication Guide for Fluoroquinolone Antibiotics.* Wayne, NJ: Bayer Healthcare Pharmaceuticals, Inc. 2013.

8. "New Fluoroquinolone Warning Label." *Journal of the American Medical Association* 1996; 276:774.

9. Melhus, A. "Fluoroquinolones and Tendon Disorders." *Expert Opinion on Drug Safety* 2005; 4(2):2993-09.

10. Kim, GK, Del Rosso, JQ. "The Risk of Fluoroquinolone-Induced Tendinopathy and Tendon Rupture: What does the clinician need to know?" *Journal of Clinical and Aesthetic Dermatology* 2010, 3(41) 49-54.

11. Williams, RJ, Attia, E, Wickiewicz, TW, Hannafin, JA. "The Effect of Ciprofloxacin on Tendon, Paratendon, and Capsular Fibroblast Metabolism." *American Journal of Sports Medicine* 2000, 28(3):364-69.

12. Kaleagasioglu, F, Olcay, E. "Fluoroquinolone-Induced Tendinopathy: Etiology and Preventative Measures." *Tohoku Journal of Experimental Medicine* 2012, 226:251-58.

13. Adikwu, E, Brambaifa, N." Ciprofloxacin-Induced Chondrotoxicity and Tendinopathy." *American Journal of Pharmacology and Toxicology* 2012, 7(3):94-100.

14. Tsai, WC, Yang, YM. "Fluoroquinolone Associated Tendinopathy." *Chang Gung Medical Journal* 2011, 34(5):461-67.

15. Khaliq, Y, Zhanel, GG. "Musculoskeletal Injury Associated with Fluoroquinolone Antibiotics." *Clinical Plastic Surgery* 2005, 32(4):495-50.

16. Gürbay, A, Gonthier, B, Signorini-Allibe, N, et al. "Ciprofloxacin Induced DNA Damage in Primary Culture of Rat Astrocytes and Protection by Vitamin E." *Neurotoxicology* 2006, 27(1):6-10.

17. Corps, AN, Harrall, RL, Curry, VA, et al. "Ciprofloxacin Enhances the Stimulation of Matrix Metalloproteinase 3 Expression by Interleukin-1beta in Human Tendon Derived Cells: A Potential Mechanism of Fluoroquinolone Induced Tendinopathy?" *Arthritis and Rheumatism* 2002, 46(11):3034-40.

18. Pouzaud, F, Bernard-Beaubois, K, Thevenin, M, et al. "Vitro Disinhibition of Fluoroquinolones Toxicity on Tendon Cells: Involvement of Oxidative Stress." *Journal of Pharmacology and Experimental Therapeutics* 2003, 308(1)394-402.

19. Shakibaei, M, de Souza, P, van Sickle, D, Stahlmann, R. "Biochemical Changes in Achilles Tendon from Juvenile Dogs After Treatment with Ciprofloxacin or Feeding a Magnesium-Deficient Diet." *Archives of Toxicology* 2001, 75(6)369-74.

20. Biundo, JJ, Mipro, RC, Fahey, P. "Sports Related and Other Soft Tissue Injuries, Tendinitis, Bursitis, and Occupation Related Syndromes." *Current Opinion in Rheumatology* 1997, 9(2):151-54.

21. *Physicians' Desk Reference,* 62nd Ed. Montvale, NJ: Medical Economics Company, 2008.

22. van der Linden, PD, Sturkenboom, MC, Herings, RM, et al. "Increased Risk of Achilles Tendon Rupture with Quinolone Antibacterial Use, Especially in Elderly Patients Taking Corticosteroids." *Archives of Internal Medicine* 2003, 163:1801-7.

23.Sendzik, J, Lode, H, Stahlmann J. "Quinolone-Induced Arthropathy: An Update Focusing on New Mechanistic and Clinical Data." *International Journal of Antimicrobial Agents* 2009, 33(3):194-200.

24. Polacheck, H, Leibovitz, E, Dagan, R. "Joint Cartilage Lesions Caused by Quinolones in Young Animals: Can We Generalize to Children?" *Harefuah* 2011, 150(9):721-upright 24, 750.

25. Committee on Infectious Diseases. "The Use of Systemic Fluoroquinolones." *Pediatrics* 2006, 118(3):1287-92.

26. Forsythe, CT, Ernst, ME. "Do Fluoroquinolones Commonly Cause Arthropathy in Children?" *Canadian Journal of Emergency Medicine* 2007, 9(6)459-62.

27. Rosanova, MT, Lede, R, Capurro, H, et al. "Assessing Fluoroquinolones as Risk

Factor for Musculoskeletal Disorders in Children: A Systematic Review and Meta-analysis." *Archives of Argentina Pediatrics* 2010, 108(6):524-31.

28. Noel, GJ, Bradley, JS, Kauffman, RE, et al. "Comparative Safety Profile of Levofloxacin in 2,523 Children with a Focus on Four Specific Musculoskeletal Disorders." *Pediatric and Infectious Disease* 2007, 26(10)879-91.

29. Chalmeau, M, et al. "Fluoroquinolone Safety in Pediatric Patients: A Prospective, Multicenter, Comparative Cohort Study in France." *Pediatrics* 2003, 111(6) 714-19.

30. Stahlmann, C. "Children as a Special Population at Risk: Quinolones as an Example for Xenobiotics Exhibiting Skeletal Toxicity." *Archives of Toxicology* 2003, 77(1)771.

Chapter 3. Toxicity in the Central and Peripheral Nervous Systems

1. Galland, MC, Jouve-Bestange , MH, et al. "Neurologic Side Effects of Quinolones." *Therapie* 1982; 4817.

2. "Therapy of Acute and Chronic Gramnegative Osteomyelitis with Ciprofloxacin." *Journal of Antimicrobial Chemotherapy* 1988; 2218.

3. Aoun, M, Jacquy, C, Debusscher, D, et al. "Peripheral Neuropathy Associated with Fluoroquinolones." *Lancet* 1992, 127.

4. Hedenmalm, K, Spigset, O. "Peripheral Sensory Disturbances Related to Treatment with Fluoroquinolones." *Journal of Antimicrobial Chemotherapy* 1996, 37(4):8317.

5. Cohen, JS. "Peripheral Neuropathy Associated with Fluoroquinolone Antibiotics." *Annals of Pharmacotherapy* 2001, 35(12):1540-47

6. U.S. Food and Drug Administration, Safety Announcement, August 8, 2013.

7. *Medical Letter on Drugs and Therapeutics* 2013; 89.

8. *Physicians' Desk Reference,* 66th Ed., Montvale NJ: Medical Economics Company, 2012.

9. Slavich, IL, Gleffe, RF, Haas, EJ. "Grand mal Epileptic Seizures During Ciprofloxacin Therapy." *Journal of the American Medical Association* 1989; 261(4):5589.

10. Bellon, A, Perez-Garcia, G, Coverdale, JH, Chacko RC. "Seizures Associated with Levofloxacin: Case Presentation and Literature Review." *European Journal of Clinical Pharmacology* 2009, 65(10):959-62

11. Darwish, T. "Ciprofloxacin-Induced Seizures in a Healthy Patient." *New Zealand Medical Journal* 2008; 121(1277):104-105.

12. Orr, CF, Rowe, DB. "Eardrop Attacks: Seizures Triggered by Ciprofloxacin Eardrops." *Medical Journal Australia* 2003, 178(7):343.

Chapter 4. Toxicity in the Brain, Heart, and Gut

1. "Clostridium Difficile Infection." Centers for Disease Control and Prevention, www.cdc.gov/hai/organisms/cdiff/cdiff_infect.html.

2. Adikwu, E, Brambaifa, N. "Ciprofloxacin Cardiotoxicity and Hepatoxicity in Humans and Animals." *Pharmacology and Pharmacy* 2012; 3(2):207-213.

3. Rubenstein, E, Camm, J. "Cardiotoxicity of Fluoroquinolones". *Journal of Antimicrobial Chemotherapy* 2002, 49:593-596.

4. Doussau, A, de Bazingan, et al. "Psychiatric Adverse Effects of Fluoroquinolone: Review of Cases from the French Pharmacologic Surveillance Database." *Review of Internal Medicine* 2006, 27(6)448-52.

Chapter 5. Do Quinolones Damage Human DNA?

1. Ronald, R, Low, DE. "Fluoroquinolone Antibiotics." Basel, Switzerland: Birkhauser Verlag, 2003.

2. Bromberg, KD, Burgin, AB, Osheroff, N. "Quinolone Action Against Human Topoisomerase II alpha: Stimulation of enzyme-mediated double stranded DNA cleavage." *Biochemistry* 2003, 42(12):3393-3398.

3. Adikwu, E. *Pharmacology and Pharmacy 2012*, 3:207-213.

4. King, J. "Fluoroquinolone DNA Testing Project Results." 2014.

5. Ambulkar, PS, Ghosh, SK, Ingole, IV, Pal, AK. "Genotoxic and Cytotoxic Effects of Antibacterial Drug, Ciprofloxacin, on Human Lymphocytes in Vitro." *Nepal Medical College Journal* 2009, 11(3): 147-151.

6. Gürbay, A, Gonthier, B, Daveloose, O, et al. "Microsomal Metabolism of Ciprofloxacin Generates Free Radicals." *Free Radical Biology and Medicine* 2001, 30(10): 1118-1121.

Chapter 6. The Benefits of Magnesium

1. Cohen, JS. "Peripheral Neuropathy Associated with Fluoroquinolone Antibiotics." *Annals of Pharmacotherapy* 2001; 1540-1547.

2. Curriculum Vitae: In Memory of Dr. Mildred Seelig 1920-2005. Center for Magnesium Education and Research, magnesiumeducation.com/about-us.

3. Stahlmann, R, Förster, M, Shakibaei, M, Vormann, et al. "Magnesium Deficiency Induces Joint Cartilege Lesions in Juvenile Rats Which Are Identical to Quinolone-Induced Arthropathy." *Antimicrobial Agents and Chemotherapy* 1995, 39(9):2013-2018.

4. Förster, C, Kociok, K, Shakibaei, M, et al. "Integrins on Joint Cartilege Chondrocytes and Alterations by Ofloxacin or Magnesium Deficiency in Immature Rats." *Archives of Toxicology* 1996, 70(5):261-270.

5. Günther, T, Rücker, M, Förster, et al. "In Vitro Evidence for a Donnan Distribution of Mg2+ and Ca2+ by Chronroitin Sulphate in Cartilage." *Archives of Toxicology* 1997, 71(7):471-475.

6. Walter, I, Egerbacher, M, Wolfesberger, B, Sieberl, G. "Confocal Laser Scanning Microscopy of Chrondocytes in Vitro: Cytoskeletal Changes After Quinolone Treatment." *Scanning* 1998; 511-15.

7. Stahlmann, R, Lode, H. "Toxicity of Quinolones." *Drugs* 1999; 37-42.

8. Shakibaei ,M, Pfister, K, Schwabe, R, Vormann, J, Stahlmann, R. "Ultrastructure

of Achilles Tendons of Rats Treated with Ofloxacin and Fed a Normal or Magnesium-Deficient Diet." *Antimicrobial Agents and Chemotherapy* 2000, 44(2)261-266.

9. Shakibei, M, de Souza, P, van Sickle, D, Stahlmann, R. "Biochemical Changes in Achilles Tendons from Juvenile Dogs After Treatment with Ciprofloxacin or Feeding a Magnesium Deficient Diet." *Archives of Toxicology* 2001, 75(6):369-374.

10. Kushner, JM, Peckman, HJ, Snyder, CR. "Seizures Associated with Fluoroquinolones." *Annals of Pharmacotherapy* 2001, 35: 1194-1198.

11. Lozo, E, Riecke, K, Schwave, R, et al. "Synergistic Effects of Ofloxacin and Magnesium Deficiency on Joint Cartilage in Immature Rats." *Antimicrobial Agents in Chemotherapy* 2002, 46(6) 1755-1759.

12. Stahlmann R, Förster, C, Shakibaei, M, Vormann, J, Günther, T, and Murker, H. "Magnesium Deficiency Induces Joint Cartilage Lesions in Juvenile Rats Which Are Identical to Quinolone-Induced Arithropathy." *Antimicrobial Agents and Chemotherapy* 1995.

13. Shakibei, M, de souza, P, van Sickle, D, Stahlmann, R. "Biochemical Changes in Achilles Tendon from Juvenile Dogs." *Archives of Toxicology* 2001, 75(6):369-374.

14. Pfister, K, Mazur, D, Vormann, J, Stahlmann, R. "Diminished Ciprofloxacin-Induced Chrondotoxicity by Supplementation with Magnesium and Vitamin E in Immature Rats." *Antimicrobial Agents and Chemotherapy* 2007, 51(3): 1022-1027. 8 January 2007.

15. U.S. Food and Drug Administration. "FDA Drug Safety Communication: Low Magnesium Levels Can Be Associated with Long-Term Use of Proton Pump Inhibitor Drugs (PPIs)." FDA Safety Announcement, 2 March 2011.

16. Johnson, RD, Dorr, MB, Talbot, GH. "Effect of Maalox on the Oral Absorption of Sparfloxacin." *Clinical Therapeutics* 1998; 20(6): 1149-1158.

Chapter 7. The Benefits of N-Acetylcysteine, Zinc, and Vitamin E

1. Kalghatgi, S. et al. "Bactericidal Antibiotics Induce Mitochondrial Dysfunction and Oxidative Damage in Mammalian Cells." *Science Translational* Medicine 2013; 5:192.

2. Natural Medicines: The Authority on Integrative Medicine. "Nature Medicine Quality Standards." 2014. naturalmedicines.therapeuticresearch.com.

3. Kalghatgi et al. "Bactericidal Antibiotics Induce Mitochondrial Dysfunction and Oxidative Damage in Mammalian Cells." *Science Translational Medicine* 2013, 5:192.

4. Pfister, K, Mazur, D, Vormann, J, Stahlmann, R. "Diminished Ciprofloxacin-Induced Chrondotoxicity by Supplementation with Magnesium and Vitamin E in Immature Rats." *Antimicrobial Agents and Chemotherapy* 2007, 51(3):1022-1027. 8 January 2007.

5. Gürbay, A, Gonthier, B, Signorini-Allibe, N, et al. "Ciprofloxacin-Induced DNA Damage in Primary Culture of Rat Astrocytes and Protection by Vitamin E." *Neurotoxicology* 2006, 27:6-10.

6. Gürbay, A, Gontheir, B, et al. "Microsmal Metabolism of Ciprofloxacin and Tendinopathy." *American Journal of Pharmacology and Toxicology* 2012, 7(3):94-100.

7. Channa, HM, Ashfaq, M, Bangash, R, et al. "Preventative Role of Zinc Chloride Against Toxicity of Ciprofloxacin on the Growing Cartilage of Wistar Albino Rat Litter." *Journal of Ayub Medical College* 2008, 20(4):77-81.

Chapter 8, Tried and True Remedies

1. Lasser, KE, Allen, PD, Woolhandler, SJ, et al. "Timing of New Black Box Warnings and Withdrawals for Prescription Medications." *Journal of the American Medical Association* 2002, 287:20.

2. Cipro package insert. Bayer Healthcare Pharmaceuticals, Wayne, NJ: 2008.

3. Guyatt, G, Rennie, D. *Guide to the Medical Literature: A Manual for Evidence-Based Clinical Practice.* Chicago: American Medical Association, 2002.

2. Natural Medicines: The Authority on Integrative Medicine. "Nature Medicine Quality Standards." 2014. naturalmedicines.therapeuticresearch.com.

5. Wernicke, J, Dunlop, S, Dornseif, B, Bosomworth, J, Humbert, M. "Low Dose, Fluoxetine Therapy for Depression." *Psychopharmacology Bulletin* 1998, 24(1):183-188.

6. Hal, MM, Finoff, JT, Smith, J. "Musculoskeletal Complications of Fluoroquinolones; Guidelines and Precautions for Usage in the Athletic Population." *Physical Medicine and Rehabilitation* 2011, 3:2:132-142.

7. Greene, BL. "Physical Therapist Management of Fluoroquinolone-Induced Achilles Tendinopathy." *Physical Therapy* 2002, 82(12):1224-31.

8. Weiler, JM, et al. "Effects of Fexofenadine, Diphenhydramine, and in the Iowa Driving Simulator." *Annals of Internal Medicine* 2000, 132(5):354-363.

9. Marcone, P. "Generate Fresh Mitochondria with PQQ: Scientists Discover the Other COQ10." *Life Extension Magazine* 2011.

10. Teitelbaum, JE, Johnson, C, St. Cyr, J. "The Use of D-Ribose in Chronic Fatigue Syndrome and Fibromyalgia: A Pilot Study." *Journal of Alternative and Complementary* 2006, 12:857-862.

Chapter 9, What We Must Do Now

1. Cohen, JS. *Over Dose: The Case Against the Drug Companies: Prescription Drugs, Side Effects, and Your Health.* New York: Tarcher/Putnam, 2001.

2. Brody, JE. "Popular Antibiotics May Carry Serious Side Effects." *New York Times.* 10 September 2012.

3. Davidson, I. "Pays to Read the Warnings When You Open Up a Prescription." *Washington Post.* 5 August 2015.

Conclusion

1. Search FDA Adverse Events Databases: Medicines (MedWatch/AERS/FAERS), Medical Devices (MAUDE), or Vaccines (VAERS). 15 December 2014. FDAble.com

2. Melmon, KI, Morelli, HF, Hoffman, BB, Nierenberg, DW. *Melmon and Morelli's Clinical Pharmacology: Basic Principles in Therapeutics*, 3rd Ed. New York: McGraw-Hill, 1993.

3. Cullen, DJ, Bates, DW, Small, SD, et al. "The incident reporting system does not detect adverse drug events: a problem for quality improvement." *Joint Commission Journal on Quality Improvement* 1993, 21(10):5418.

4. Bates, DW. "Drugs and Adverse Drug Reactions: How Worried Should We Be?" *Journal of the American Medical Association* 1998, 279(15):1216-17.

5. Faich, GA. "Adverse Drug Reaction Monitoring." *New England Journal of Medicine* 314(1986):1589-92.

6. Dickinson, JG. "FDA Seeks to Double Effort on Confusing Drug Names." *Dickinson's FDA Review* 2000, 7(3) 13-14.

7. Scott, HD, Thacher-Renshaw A, Rosenbaum SE, et al. "Physician Reporting of Adverse Drug Reactions: Results of the Rhode Island Adverse Drug Reaction Reporting Project." *Journal of the American Medical Association* 1990, 263(13)1785-88.

8. Moore, TJ. "Understanding FDA adverse event reports: guide to interpreting adverse events reports." U.S. Food and Drug Administration.

9. George, CF. "Adverse Drug Reactions and Secrecy." *British Medical Journal* 304(1992):1328.

10. Morris, LA. "A Survey of Patients' Receipt of Prescription Drug Information." *Medical Care* 20, 1982(6)596-605.

11. Braddock, CH, Edwards, KA, Hasengerb, NM, et al. "Informed decision making in outpatient practice: Time to get back to basics." *Journal of the American Medical Association* 1999, 282: 2313-20.

12. Braddock, CH, Fihn, SD, Levinson, W, et al. "How doctors and patients discuss routine clinical decisions: Informed decision making in the outpatient setting." *Journal of General Internal Medicine* 1997, 12(6)339-45.

13. Frieden, T. "Antibiotic prescribing in hospitals: improvement needed." Medscape. 4 March 2014. www.medscape.com/viewarticle/821135?nlid=51084_491&src=wnl_edit_medp_wir& uac=120412AX&spon=17.

14. Linder, JA, Stafford, S. "Antibiotic treatment of liberal with sore drug by humidity primary care physicians: A National Survey, 1989-1999." *Journal of the American Medical Association* 2001, 286(10)1181-86.

About the Author

Jay S. Cohen, M.D., is a nationally respected expert on prescription medications and side effects, a driving force for the implementation of better methods to reduce the high rate of medication-related deaths (150,000) and hospitalizations (2,000,000) annually in America. He is also an expert on natural remedies.

Dr. Cohen earned his medical degree at Temple University, Philadelphia, in 1971. After completing his internship, he practiced general medicine and subsequently conducted ground-breaking research at UCLA in 1973 on acupuncture and pain. In 1974, he undertook a residency in psychiatry and psychopharmacology at the University of California, San Diego. He has been an associate adjunct professor of preventative and family medicine, psychiatry, and medication safety at UCSD for many decades. He is also the Chairman of the Medical Advisory Committee of the Erythromelalgia Association, as well as a Fellow of the American College of Nutrition.

The emphasis of Dr. Cohen's work has been on prevention. He has performed independent research in pharmacology, specifically on the causes of medication side effects. Dr. Cohen's identification of a substantial portion of the population that is medication-sensitive has been ground-breaking. His books and articles have been featured in newspapers and magazines across America, including the *New York Times, Wall Street Journal*, and *Women's Day*. He has also appeared on hundreds of radio programs, including National Public Radio and the People's Pharmacy. His book, *Over Dose: The Case Against the Drug Companies* (Tarcher/Putnam 2001), received unanimously excellent reviews from Publishers Weekly, Library Journal, and the *Journal of the Medical American Association*.

Dr. Cohen has been the keynote speaker at major medical conferences and debated top FDA officials on drug safety. His work has been unique in informing people around the world about serious problems in the pharmaceutical and medical industry, and how people can use mediations more safely and effectively. He now informs us about the terrible harm that has come to tens of thousands of patients from toxic antibiotics like Cipro and Levaquin, and what we can do to protect ourselves and our families—even when the drugs are necessary!

Dr. Cohen conducts his research, writing, and office practices in Del Mar, California.

Index

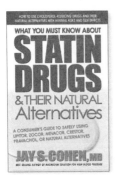

What You Must Know About Statin Drugs & Their Natural Alternatives
Jay S. Cohen, MD

Over 20 million Americans take statin drugs to treat their high cholesterol levels. This guide explains how to use statins with minimal risk of side effects, and also highlights natural cholesterol-lowering remedies and key nutrients for cardiovascular health.

$15.95 US • 224 pages • 6 x 9-inch paperback • ISBN 978-0-7570-0257-1

Natural Alternatives to Lipitor, Zocor & Other Statin Drugs
Jay S. Cohen, MD

Statins are a class of drugs used to treat high cholesterol and inflammation, but nearly half of those who take them experience side effects. This guide explains the problems caused by statins and provides effective natural alternatives.

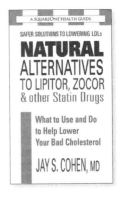

$7.95 US • 144 pages • 4 x 7-inch paperback • ISBN 978-0-7570-0286-1

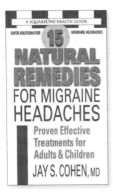

15 Natural Remedies for Migraine Headaches
Jay S. Cohen, MD

For anyone who has yet to find relief from migraines, best-selling author Jay Cohen offers a concise, comprehensive, and practical guide to natural remedies that are just as effective as their conventional counterparts, but much safer.

$7.95 US • 160 pages • 4 x 7-inch paperback • ISBN 978-0-7570-0358-5

Unsafe at Any Meal

Dr. Renee Joy Dufault

Each year, Americans consume hundreds of food products that contain dangerous compounds, including heavy metals, pesticides, and harmful additives. Why haven't we heard about this? In *Unsafe at Any Meal*, Dr. Renee Dufault, former food investigator for the Food and Drug Administration, provides the startling answers. Dr. Dufault also presents an in-depth look at the toxic substances commonly found in our food supply and explains how they affect our genes, our health, and the surrounding environment. Backed by research and first-hand experience, Dr. Dufault reveals how the FDA has failed us, and outlines how you can protect yourself and your family by knowing which foods to avoid.

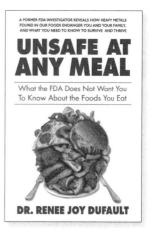

$16.95 US • 240 pages • 6 x 9-inch paperback •
ISBN 978-0-7570-0436-0

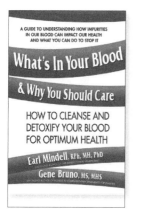

What's In Your Blood & Why You Should Care

Earl Mindell, RPh, MH, PhD, and Gene Bruno, Ms, MHS

Like most people, you probably get a blood test and keep your fingers crossed until the results come back. But while these tests focus on key components of your blood, they provide only a limited view of what's going on inside you. Blood tests don't tell you about heavy metals or unwanted pathogens that may be coursing through your body. *What's In Your Blood & Why You Should Care* is the first book to provide a complete picture of the components that make up your blood, how it functions, and what you can do to improve its quality for greater health and longevity. From diets to supplements to medical treatments, it's all there in this groundbreaking book.

$16.95 US • 240 pages • 6 x 9-inch paperback •
ISBN 978-0-7570-0443-8

Turmeric for Your Health

Larry Trivieri, Jr.

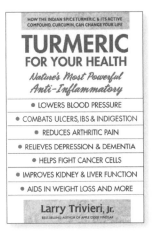

Imagine a natural spice that has the power to reduce or eliminate inflammation, the underlying cause of many serious health disorders. For over 5,000 years, India's Ayurvedic medical practitioners have used turmeric to treat a host of painful and debilitating diseases. Recently, medical researchers in the US have turned their attention to this ancient root and have discovered its effectiveness in lowering blood pressure, reducing arthritis pain, increasing brain function, combating gastrointestinal issues, aiding in weight loss, and much more. *Turmeric for Your Health* is a simple guide to understanding the science behind turmeric's effectiveness. With few if any side effects, turmeric can offer a safe, inexpensive way to enhance your health and well-being.

$15.95 US • 192 pages • 6 x 9-inch paperback • ISBN 978-0-7570-0452-0

Coconuts for Your Health

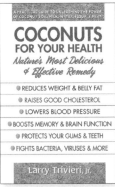

Larry Trivieri, Jr.

Before their introduction to the Standard Western Diet, natives of the South Pacific islands were among the healthiest people in the world. Heart disease and obesity were extremely rare, as were infectious diseases, dementia, and dental issues. Remarkably, the majority of calories consumed by the islanders came from coconuts. Today, medical researchers have rediscovered the many health benefits of this tropical fruit. Coconut has been found to raise good cholesterol, reduce belly fat, boost memory, protect teeth and gums, lower blood pressure, and more. This book focuses on specific concerns from heart disease to high blood pressure to memory loss, and explains how coconut works to combat these issues.

$15.95 US • 208 pages • 6 x 9-inch paperback • ISBN 978-0-7570-0451-3

31901063241725

**For more information about our books,
visit our website at www.squareonepublishers.com**